For Chris,

In celebration of
daring to connect and freeing
to tears.   With love and grace,

~ Jamie
3.13.19

BEDSIDE PORTRAITS

ON HOSPICE TIME

Janine Carranza, RN

First Edition

ISBN 978-0-692-19320-4

Printed by Ingram Sparks

Jacket Design & Book Cover
by Anya Katrina Smith

Jacket Art (back cover), © Kate Frothingham

Editor - Cecelia Hagan

Cover Photo:

Besty Eckfeldt returned from her last visit to her son
and needed to sit before reaching her bed.

Chapter Titles:

The Seven Valleys by Bahá'u'lláh

Contributing Poets:

Kim Bakondi

Mary Brutsaert

Robert Daley Jr

Mary Ellis

Rachel Houck

Troy Maddux

(Henry Scott-Holland)

David Whyte

Christian Wiman

Scott Wilson

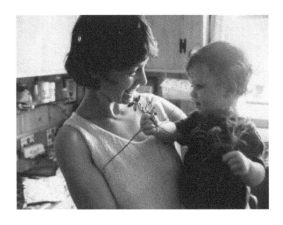

Para Mi Papá Que Me Leyó Cuentos de Niña a Mujer

Para Mi Hermano Todd, My Best Friend and Confidant of a Lifetime.

For the Dead Who Keep Us Company.
And For My Daughters Who Teach Me the World of Mystery.

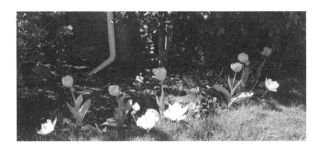

Tulips planted by *Señorito Pepito* in 2014

The names of the patients and families in this book are changed, to honor their privacy. It has been hard to change the names of those to whom I am endeared, and to whom the stories belong. Colleagues and family have opted to allow their names to stand. To all I have attempted to do justice, if that is possible, with these people who are my world — our world.

The way to love anything

is to realize that it might be lost.

In life, the currency we trade

to show what we value most, is time.

Money comes and goes,

but time is the most limited commodity we have.

Consciously or unconsciously,

our action and devotion to ourselves,

others and our skills and crafts which we pursue

are a direct reflection of what we consider valuable.

If we had forever, it would dilute what is really special.

In many ways, mortality is a gift.

~ Anonymous

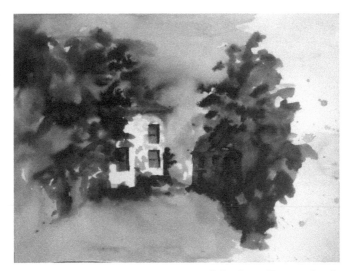

CONTENTS

The Valley of Knowledge

The Valley of Unity

The Valley of Contentment

The Valley of Wonderment

The Valley of True Poverty and Absolute Nothingness

A NOTE FROM THE AUTHOR

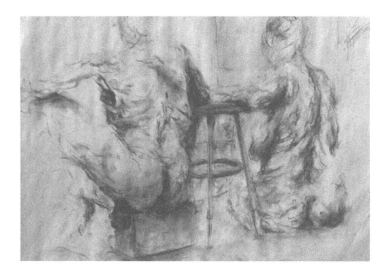

The closing chapter of a life is not the one some of us grew up with where we think death is frightening, as a freakish inability to breathe or exist. It is the reality of the last breath of release from the bondage of the attached, into an expansive unknown.

It is not the death of everything that we hold dear, but the welcoming into what is most precious in life. It is the loss of our earthly physical companions, expanded into the deepest connection of one to another forever. Hospice has taught me that the sense of separation is something imagined from our humanly hesitations. It is clear from this work that we are together, not separate. It is clear that we must express our bond in whatever way we find, especially at death when the greatest fear is the opposite: loss of connection.

Spirits have known this for centuries. The dying speak this voice. Those who listen, hear the same. When you read their cries, know that no detail in these portraits is invented or altered but through the filter of my perception.

I remember as a young girl watching the candle lit in my room in Mexico where we did not have electricity. It seemed to me that the candle was a life, maybe my life. When I watched it, it seemed to go on forever. But when I woke up in the morning, the flame and most of the wax was gone; it was extinguished with few remains visible. Would that be my life? My family's life? What in the wick that lay small and black at the bottom of the glass would remain? Anything? Nothing? Was the flame gone forever? In thin air? What did Nothing mean? I would try to conceive of *nothing*, and it scared me to the core as a little girl: Nothing ? ?

It is the same question that comes to us when we die: In millisecond review, or in a longer reflective period if we get that privilege, we are flooded with pressing questions: *"Am I leaving anything lasting behind? Was it all worth it? Was any of it worth it? How am I leaving my loved ones behind? Will they be okay? Am I needed anymore? Was I ever needed? Did I love enough? Did I laugh enough? Did I remember what counts and not get lost in the distraction of what doesn't count for very long?"* Or: *"For the times that I did forget the important, did I then regain my priorities? Have I reconciled what I can with the people I love? Am I where I want to be in my life now? Do I... did I... Matter?"* And, of course: *"Where am I going? Anywhere? Will it hurt? Will it stop hurting? Will there be any continuation? Or none at all? Will it be scary? Will anyone come to meet me? Will I remain connected?"*

I remember coming across the border into the U.S.A. at eleven years old for the first time on Christmas Eve. Texas loomed in expansiveness and emptiness that confused my spirit. Where was the music, where were the people and smells and children and fireworks and dogs scrounging for scraps? I saw nothing of the hearths that are now my world. Only the emptiness that in Mexico is so full.

In the years of growing up as a young adult in North America, I could not find my Mexican grandmother in the streets, walking to the market, and giving consolation to the people who were hurting. I did not understand the role of elders in the nursing homes here. I didn't understand why my great, great grand aunt from the North American side of my family — Eva, the first woman who graduated from Yale Divinity School — was in a nursing home where no one wanted to play *Scrabble* with her persistently active mind. I wanted her to live with me, but didn't have a home into which I could bring her. The long streets without town centers like the Mexican Zócalo, the bandstand and promenade. The city planning and architectural design, with parking coming before the pedestrian and community experience, made it feel to me a world of ghosts without family. Something was wrong in my new world.

And something was right. I got the opportunity of higher education. The opportunity of being seen as an equal as a woman. The opportunity to dream and develop without overt cultural restraint. As I found my feet and voice, after half of a century feeling misunderstood in a foreign culture, I have now been welcomed and met, and given a place at the table.

My liberal arts education at Earlham College, felt rich in the intellectual realm, but also wanting in the realm of the tangible. I took leaves of absence from college to live with my dad in Mexico who started schools for children who did not have access to education. When I had come to North America, Dad had stayed in Mexico. I missed him. When we were together we nursed people who did not have or could not afford doctors. Dad's schools taught the arts and practical skills for the students to take back to their families and hometowns.

These families and hometowns needed the youth as strong workhands. It was a huge sacrifice to allow their children to be educated since they might be enticed far away from home instead of come back to help. Dad and I would take eight- or ten-hour hikes carrying our boarding school photo albums into unknown territory to find children living on isolated goat farms in the mountains of the *Sierra Madre*. Dad wanted them to get an education that they could take back to use and improve their worlds.

That meant environmental education, farm and gardening experience, learning about the arts and literature, communication, health, community organization. It confused the townfolks' prejudices to have *Huichole* Indian children perform gloriously in concerts and theatrical plays, when it was common knowledge that the Indians did not have intelligence, social allure or charm. Often these young people did not, in fact (to Dad's great disappointment) return as locals to their home towns. But it is what Dad wished of his students.

Dad gave his life to the need at hand. I watched him enter people's worlds. He was an intuitive. He knew, not only how to introduce the mystery of the literary world with illiterate town people, how to tease, laugh with, and offer ease to a suffering being, but also how to diagnose health issues, find the vein for an IV with impossibly dehydrated, invisible, and old slippery vessels. He knew how to help people feel better.

At the age of twenty-six, I realized I had to be a nurse. My mom wanted me to be a graphic artist, or another career more visibly gallant than the hard labor of nursing. But I knew that I had to find my grandmother on my Mexican side, and that my father was passing on a gift to me. My mother helped me financially to get into nursing school. When I was done with my textbooks, I sent them to my dad. He learned from them. My brother became a doctor and did the same. My visits to Mexico over the years gave me the grounding that I needed to find my way in this foreign country north of the border. My father, my grandmother, and my brother are my spearhead teachers.

Today, when I walk into a home where someone is dying, I do not know what is ahead of me. When I leave, I don't know what happened — except for what I missed or where I erred (in hindsight) helping me to improve for my next visit. The momentary answers I find are in part from knowledge and scientific study, part guidance from my ancestors, and part the kind of experience that risks going into the world that has not yet become "evidenced-based practice" –because it is in the process of becoming so.

I have learned that following "evidence-based practice" is missing critical components. It has become the go-to safe path in the practice of Western medicine because it offers some level of reliability in some level of results, but it is missing in what is yet un-evidenced from improved results. The methods and formulas of documented practice are only as good as what has been evidenced so far. It is our job as medical professionals to carry medicine and healing to the next step, not to incessantly repeat the model practice of the last step with its incomplete results. The practice of healing will always be incomplete. It will always be growing, as long as we remain open. Vulnerability and the unknown must not be eliminated in building the model framework.

Professional vulnerability and inventiveness from educated experience, openness to grace and inspiration, is the source, not the weakness of the path.

The most important answers stem from *new* information in each visit from people we have just met, who humble and expose themselves in one of the hardest times of their lives and allow connection to happen in the face of a deteriorating body (which is every one of our bodies). Their exposure comes at a time of the greatest fear: cessation of connection to their life by death. A deteriorating body is a threat to remaining connected to what matters to us most. Whatever matters to us most, losing body function feels like losing life function.

Not so. That is the hospice lesson: Life is bigger than what our bodies encompass.

The longer you practice medicine and healing, the more brand new you need to make your next patient visit. It is our job as medical professionals to allow the sick person to lead. They know more than we do. We are but facilitators toward a body and spirit that already knows its path, yet may be stuck in places. Help un-stick. But do not be the primary orchestrator. We are not the conductor. Nor the musical instrument. It is someone else's passage. The health professional inspires and offers direction as a loving, listening companion, to help release the patient's song. The song is from the patient and their family. We are but a part of that. Even as a team of professionals, we are still small to the wholeness of a full life. Questions matter, answers may or may not come, being there is everything.

Ultimately, after the skilled medical interventions of expertly practiced hospice comfort care, there is only one thing that relieves suffering and enters the world of Mystery. It is people's realized capacity to enter into each other's existence.

This awareness helps us to know how to practice medicine that fits the patient, not fit the patient into the practice that we know in medicine. Opening takes priority to defining. Defining comes after listening and hearing. Diagnosing is limited, questioning is unlimited. To understand is to stand under, not over.

The physical world is but a metaphor to the spiritual world. In hospice, a lot of what we hear comes from symbolic language: *"I want to go home"* has many meanings to a dying person — not all based on this planet. Wanting to get out of bed when you have become bedfast, and wanting to move around when you have spent your life active, is a message of the desire and need for activity at a time when physical activity is severely limited. The agitation may not need medicating, but instead may need movement. Silence and minimal responsiveness in the last hours or days may not indicate the suffering and prolonged death that loved ones fear, but a private time to come to terms with one's life, on one's own terms. Talking on your deathbed to people who are long gone from this world may not be hallucinations of a mind going awry, but an insight into a world that we don't understand.

The art of learning to hear someone from the inside instead of the outside, without imposing personal prejudices, is the art of understanding. I think people need and deserve to be seen for who they are, not for who they aren't. When we do that, we love everyone we meet — however small that meeting of hearts is. A small connection is a big love. This completes the incomplete. When we don't understand, being there wanting to, is enough.

The perception is that the work of hospice must be hard. It is hardest when we lose connection to the eternal. But it is also to be reminded every day of what really matters, and to work with other people who are connected and fulfilled in this work. A career in hospice is one of learning, broadening exposure, humility, and constantly facing the next unknown miracle, most particularly the unknown of the next family that opens the door to a hospice stranger, bares their soul, and opens themselves to a new connection toward their wholeness. This is life.

In hospice, as in all careers, work becomes additionally hard when systems overpower the spirit of the work. Hospice is somewhat new in our culture, and it is rapidly expanding and changing from the time it was run mostly by volunteers who did not forget heart first. Today it is working to find its way back to complete commitment of service first, and business to support the service next — not vice versa in the energy focus. We must set up a good system for both the hospice patients and the service providers. Just patient-focused, is not enough. The staff have to be placed first also, so they excel in service to the patient. Few organizations and leaders understand this.

Capitalist America sometimes goes in the reverse direction. Revitalized America understands what its multitudinous immigrants are refreshing for us from our own pilgrim heritage: Love and hard work come first. They are the core. Money is not the core, nor the bottom line. The art and the science are the bottom line. The wealth is in knowing that the best things are not in things, but in us. You and me and him and her and they and us — All of us, not just some.

Dying is not just for the poor or just for the rich, not just for the educated or just for the less educated, not just for one skin color or another, not just one gender or another, not just one nationality or another. Death meets us all, and we all meet death in one way or another, later if not sooner. All of us find peace sooner or later on our death beds.

"Life is pleasant. Death is peaceful. It's the transition that's troublesome."
~Isaac Asimov

All deaths close in peace, as peace is synonymous with the last breath. Watch one thousand people close their lives to the last moment, and you will know this no matter what whatever precedes that sacred moment. A few of us find peace years before death, a few find peace months before, some find peace weeks before, for some it is days, for some the quiet open breath is found just hours before death, and for a few tormented souls, peace is not found until the last breath. Our last breath and peace is one and the same. Our last breath will be the discovery of your ultimate peace, however that looks for you.

I wanted to call this book "Dying Like You and Me," because we are all on the same path of inevitable closure to life as we know it, but the people who have read it say that this book is about living and that the title was deceiving.

As a hospice nurse I get the practice and reward of being reminded and challenged every day to be connected to what is forever. The portraits of the people described in the next pages are to me forever. They each lived, and to me, still live. If you want to know what is eternal, ask. Then listen for the answer.

To me it came like this:

NIGHTSHIFT

It's a heavy thing,
To intrude on a sleeping building.

It pushes against the noise
That crowds by as you enter.
There's a rumbling somewhere
Muffled behind stoic walls
That retreats from weekday industry.

Crunching on crystallized moments,
You see a chair
Still loyally gazing to where a back last was seen,
And give it a twirl.

~Rachel Houck, RN

Part One

INPATIENT HOSPICE

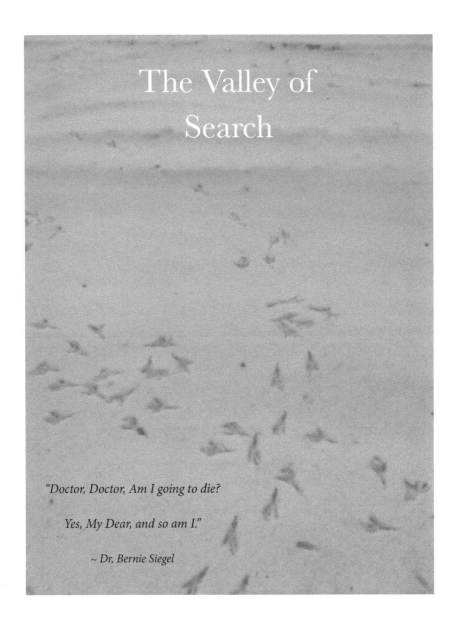

The Valley of Search

"Doctor, Doctor, Am I going to die?

Yes, My Dear, and so am I."

~ Dr, Bernie Siegel

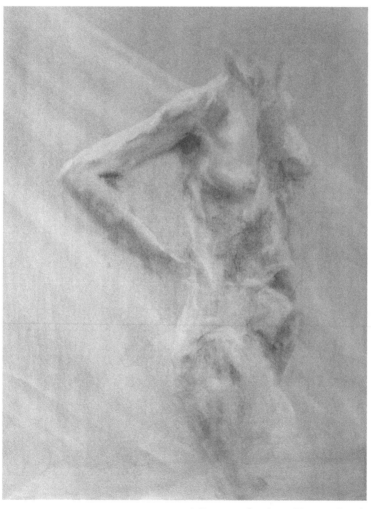

© Drawing by Anya Katrina Smith

IT'S TOO SHORT

She was the ex-wife.

"He drank all his life, and then when he was told he was going to die,
he stopped drinking.

I feel robbed. This is what we were waiting for; and now he's dying.

We were supposed to get old together.

We were supposed to get through it all and come back together again."

"You have," I said.

"But it is too short," she said.

She was sobbing and trying to hold it back.

She had just spent a week at inpatient hospice, visiting from Ohio,

and today she was going back to a new job.

"It's my first real job in thirteen years. I'm scared," she had said the night before.

"You will be great," he had said to her. *"I know it."*

"He's the best Ex- I have,"

"and I have several," her wry smile noted factually.

She kissed and caressed him.

With a wan smile broader inside, he reached out and touched her hair.

HIS BODY WAS DEAD

There was once a man, a long, thin man
with a drawn face and long fingers and feet.
His face held no color. He walked with his head slightly fallen forward.
His eyes were a very bright blue
and they looked you in the face when you saw him.

"You know," he said, *"I spent my life working at a warehouse lifting boxes.*
At one time my boss offered me a promotion. It was out-of-state.
My wife said she liked her job and my son said he didn't want to move."

He turned to look at the photo by the bedside of his wife who had died young.

"We didn't move; and they were happy." He smiled.
"Sometimes a promotion is not the best thing," he said,
"When you have what you want already."

This patient had a penectomy as part of his cancer treatment.
That was a first for me in my almost twenty years of nursing.
How does a man live through that?
He winked at me one day, *"You know, it's not that bad.*
It's not like I am dating anymore or anything."

Some people seem to find ways to make everything okay.

I wondered about this patient with his humor and burning eyes,
ready to reach out to anyone at any time, it seemed,
and how much pain he suffered quietly.
All kinds of pain.

I wondered if he felt comfortable asking for what he needed,
while he thought more about other people than his own needs.

There were times I was sure he was hurting a lot,
but when I asked him, he said he was fine.

He did, in time, let us in on his needs. He came to trust us, I think.
He was able to ask for pain medication.
At least the kind that takes away the physical pain.
And the anti-anxiety medication helped.

One day Lora, the evening nurse, walked in to see him.
His deathly paleness was ashen.
His mouth open and dry from mouth-breathing.
But there were no breaths. He was completely still.
She leaned over the face that had become dear to her.

He opened his eyes, *"April Fool's!"* he said with weak smile.
And still a slight shimmer in his eye. It was April 9th.

Twenty minutes later he was dead. At least his body was.

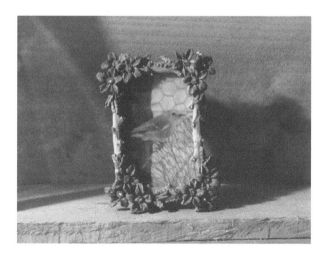

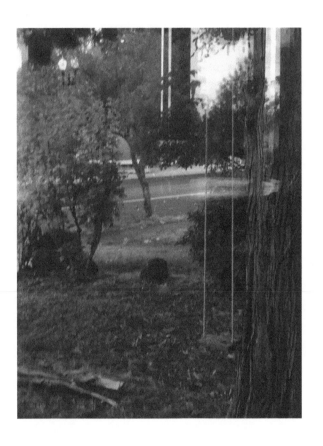

NOT DEAD

It's what I wish I could tell them:

We are all dying, and
have been most our lives, but
the fact that you can know this—that
this life is ending—means
you, you
are not dead.

You are not dead!

If you can still hear my voice,
and feel my hand in yours,
and smell the lilacs on the table,
and feel the softness of your pillow,
and see your daughter's arms 'round her daughter's arms,
and feel the rise and fall of each breath you take, then

you, you
are alive.

You are alive!

For a moment, yes
but for this moment, the only
moment that matters, the
only moment you know how
to love,
to hold,
to serenade in your own special way—the way
that makes it dance infinitum—for

this, this
is your moment.

This is your moment!

This is being alive!

I know you are dying, but
you, you
are not dead!

It's what I wish I could tell them, but,
they would never understand—at least not yet.

~ Scott Wilson, M.Div., BCC

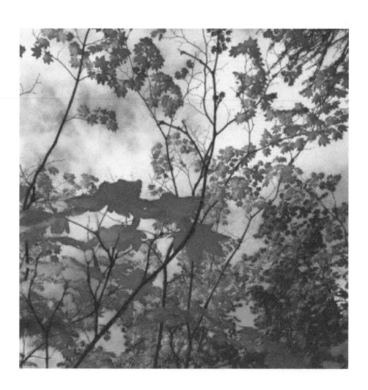

IN THE DEEPEST OF WINTER

In the deepest of winter, a bush outside the West door is filled with oblong berries so red and plentiful against the pillowed snow, that I think of fairy tales and their crisp beauty and timeless happiness. The deer look as perfect as the scene, but are on a more practical mission when food is scarce, and over time, clear the bush of any red.

Still more memorable than this is the image I have of Jackie standing feebly, with her head resting against the glass door, very close to the deer, but barred from scent-recognition. The hall is long and she looks small at the end of it, her walker in reach. I still see her. Shortly I would take her the scheduled morphine to help her breathe easy.

She was straightforward, quick to smile, slow to complain — tough and soft at the same time. I was asked to describe dying people in more physical detail, but it doesn't seem to be what I remember. Dying is about discarding the body. One succeeds in forgetting about the body with death, as a hermit crab dropping his shell, especially in the last days when it parades demise and not the prowess of life.

I now remember that Jackie was thin and bony, and I remember her telling me that she had a lot of weight on her before she got sick. It was hard to imagine. I think her hair was short and grey and straight. Her hair wasn't white. Her skin-lines were defined over her prominent skeleton. Her hands and long fingers had veins and tendons visible through the fragile skin… It was a long time ago. She was one of my very first patients when I started working five years ago at Vermont Respite House (VRH).

I remember her bright eyes. They were keen. She was ready to laugh without much effort, but she was not a jolly sort. There was something soberly honest about her. Her words were practical and clear. She had common sensibility.

She was good to the people around her. Not because her voice was sweet, or because she said kind things, but because you felt human with her; like being in the same boat on a long river and having each others back. She was one of the rare patients that stayed over a year, and was in critical condition that whole time, so could not be discharged either to home, to another facility, nor to the next world.

Jackie said she was scared that the end would be hard. She was scared of dying and not being able to breathe. I told her that the medication was very effective for relief, and that she could count on us to keep her comfortable. I was confident, being relatively new at inpatient hospice, and impressed at the effectiveness of Morphine on breath relief. But less wise, I think, in knowing that the greater forces of life are in the end not completely governed by medicine or treatments. Today I still have confidence, but more experience for the unexpected, and I am cautious about making high promises because the unknown proves always greater than any predictions.

When her time came, it was my shift. She struggled for air. I called the on-call doctor in the middle of the night, and got an order for increased morphine for her breathing, and an increased order for Lorazepam for the anxiety of air hunger. I called the doctor four times that night. She made the mistake of not giving me a high enough titration range on the first call, and I lacked the defiance to press for it.

Every fifteen minutes the nurse aide was going back and forth into Jackie's room, or the aide was staying with her and I was going back and forth, each time expecting the next doses to work. I thought I knew how to manage this.

I had promised Jackie that she would be comfortable. She didn't look comfortable. The doctor, who I thought was a pioneering queen of hospice, kept ordering just tiny increments of the medicine, without a greater range with which to work. It helped some, but I thought not enough.

The hours accumulated onto each other when minutes felt like desperacy. Jackie wasn't talking much anymore, and in a matter of hours would be unresponsive.

I was still able to ask her at one point, once again, and for the last time, "How are you doing?" Labored breathing and the experience of air hunger do not necessarily stick together, so I needed to know if she was feeling short of breath, not just looking terribly short of breath.

"I'm okay... But you don't look so good," she wheezed. I thought I was concealing my feelings better. She looking at me?

The nurse aide left at the end of his shift and, when he walked out the door, I realized how much I had been leaning on his teamship. I reached my limit of love tolerance and called my boss to cover for me. She called the doctor and got a sufficient increase in the morphine order.

I went home, and was told that Jackie died comfortably a few hours later. Her symptom management in the end was closer than it had felt. The staff and family had been with her until her last breaths.

Most memorable for me is the image of Jackie standing feebly, with her head resting against the glass door, next to the red berries and the deer.

I had asked her one day, when we still conversed in person, if she would stick around after she died and help the ones that follow her. She said with a seriousness of intent that she would. Her promise proved true.

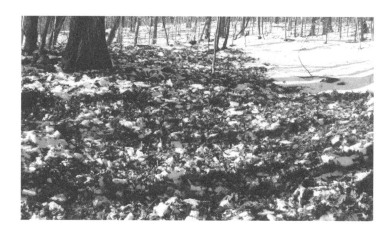

DEATH HERE

I open the door
and smell it
in the air and see it
laying on each surface like fallen snow.

Death is here.

His breath falters from
the liquid in his chest and
gurgles
back and forth
in his throat.

His mouth lays open
and the hairs on his neck
twitch,
twitch,
twitch.

His eyes are no longer
closing and the silence
screams
for words
and my heart curls up
with its hands over its ears
and screams back.

His breath quickens
and crescendos—up, up, up

and then

f

a

l

l

s

—faster
longer
farther than before.

"I am here. I love you. It's ok,"

words
echo in me,
or is it in him?
I don't know, but
I'm glad they were said `
before my heart gets the best of me.

~ Scott Wilson, M.Div., BCC

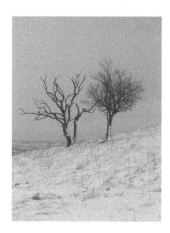

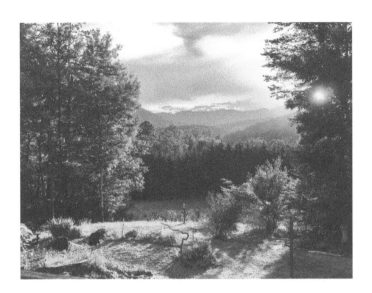

THE FARMER

Five am wide awake, a new shirt, up for the day. *"I was just fixing a broken electrical line from a fallen branch in the storm."* This morning he wasn't talking about the cows to milk.

He was happy as an inpatient resident, where we kept a close tab on his changing symptoms — because his body felt so much better with the close nursing care and treatment-plan adjustments at any time of day or night, and he didn't feel a burden to his family.

"I chose to come here. Every time I had an episode [of not being able to breathe with COPD] *it would scare me and scare my family."* His heart was still failing, his lungs still holding fluid, his legs usually puffed almost to bursting until he put them up after the latest increase of diuretic, while we watched his blood pressure and symptoms for electrolyte imbalance… What with all, he felt relatively good.

He told stories about his health and stories about his family. He flirted with the caregivers. He teased me and said he was upset that I was getting married. I told him that polygamy in some places was legal. (If somewhere that was unprofessional, with Edward it was okay.) He loved everyone. Especially his wife who had died many years ago.

He almost never said anything negative or derogatory — Until later when he started to get increasingly tired, and he increasingly lamented the old days as past. Today's new world was more than he found in him to cope.

So he held tight to his memories and started to talk about the modern world threatening the continuation of what he held dear in his life, and threatening its development in the lives of his children and grandchildren. It became too hard to bypass the challenges that crossed his family's paths. Then after he ranted about what he saw on television and how the world is not like it used to be, he was back to his contagiously jolly Edward for the next while.

I can still feel his warmth and energy as he stood in his doorway for the next passerby. His face cheered many a person's day, the staff and me included.

Hard work and diligence and manageable goals had been his ticket to success. He knew how to use an inhaler like no patient I had. I think every iota of medication would have gotten into his poor dilapidated respiratory tract, if it had anything to do with how he exhaled ahead, inhaled deeply, and held it in for as long as his breath would hold.

"I had great doctors and great nurses. I listened to what they taught me, and I did what they told me to do."

For decades he held his farm together by taking his treatments seriously and laughing a lot. Laughing was part of every shift with Edward. His face wrinkles laughed even when he was serious.

When there was little more to perfect in his daily care practice, scarce more good physical health goals, few more treatments to make him feel better — only more sleepiness and the comfort of sleep — he didn't know what to do with himself if he was awake. And it scared him.

He knew little about a life of resignation. And had not yet learned a life of letting go of the tangible. He had held his family together by the opposite: persistence and a strong grip. Dying by release over time didn't make any sense to him.

He started to retain CO2 and get confused. He could tell he was confused. Getting confused, confused him, and upset him. He began to despair. You could tell that he didn't know how to be seen despairing because he avoided talking about it under almost any conditions, even in the privacy of the trust he had developed with staff.

He hated any new faces. We tried to get volunteers to spend time with him because only sitting with him really gave him relief while he was awake. He would tell the volunteers to leave. He had energy only for the people that had already entered his circle of love. Even new caregivers became a burden with his declining energy.

Some people learn to die during life by practicing over years the art of letting go to the greater energy of things that is bigger than themselves and their own initiative. As with the two Buddhist women who practiced this in life and died their graceful deaths in the same hall in which Edward now lived. The two women were meditative, connected to the hearts of the people they love, and spent their earthly time with them.

Edward's work might have been his meditation. And spending his earthly time with the people he loved, was also his life. Still, I thought, he had little practice dying to this world. He had lived hard. And now dying was hard.

His family would visit and want to be with him. He had a lot of visitors in the daytime. Life with Edward had been good and people want to be around the good. His 7-year-old grandson made drawings of trees and brought them to him. *"He's going to make something of this one day,"* Edward would say. I bought the drawing that was framed in mahogany in the facility art gallery. It still hangs in my nurse's office: A child's touch with its shape of aged nature, in the form of a tree's trunk and branches.

On those mornings that Edward woke stressed with farm work, I told him that I had gotten up early and taken care of his cows. He sort of knew it was made-up, but it gave him permission to sleep-in when his body wanted and needed sleep.

Then Edward let go his work, he stopped fighting things, he relaxed — not from a day of physical labor, not from the good practice of his medical treatment, not even in the enjoyment of the beautiful sunny day in which he died. But with the people he had spent his life laughing and crying.

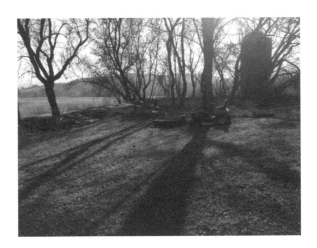

DYIN' DRY

Dyin' dry
Tears to cry
End is sly
Wonders why
Feelings shy
Sees the sky
'Bout to fly

~ Troy Maddux, LMT

WHAT

What can heal the heart,

Give rest to the scarred soul?

The longings of might-have-beens, should-have-beens,

The withering of dreams that burned you up

The painfully beautiful memories, like pressed flowers,

That no one else recalls; or treasures,

The losses of what you never had,

And the loss of what you thought would stay forever.

~Rachel Houck, RN

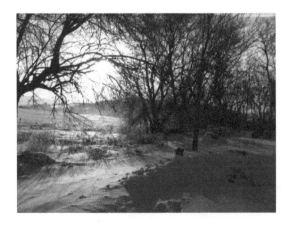

PATIENTS OR PEOPLE

She was demure.

Completely un-selfconsciously so.

She had the kind of unimaginable cancer that was not imagined. Vulvular.
Huge obtrusive tumors that consumed her pelvis. Drainage. Mess. Smell.

You couldn't see any of it in her face.
With the blankets pulled up, you could bypass the paleness of her complexion,
and the thinness of the flesh over her cheekbones.

Her smile and pleasantness made you forget she was a patient.

It's good to remember that people are people before they are patients.

And that patients are not patients, as much as people.

"You know, I couldn't give pleasure to my husband for many years.
When I found out about it, I told him that I would understand
if he wanted to leave me for a new wife. I wanted him to be happy.
But he said that he wanted to be with me — that he liked being with me."

On another night she said,

"For the last years of his life I cleaned him up
when he couldn't go to the bathroom anymore.
I washed all his clothes by hand many times a day. I didn't mind."

"Did he wear anything for padding?" I found myself compelled to ask,
when envisioning the years of days washing by hand like that,
without the incontinence products we now use,
(what with their affront to our dignity in adulthood).
"I didn't know about that stuff," she said simply.

I don't imagine she asked him for a new husband.

The day she died none of the staff had reported signs of death.
The report said there had been some pain — resolved.
She had been given morphine three times during the day —
only a little more than she usually took. An aide had called the nurse in,
saying last minute that there were changes visible despite the quiet nature
of the woman who did not draw attention to herself.
She did not show her diseased body.
Or its ending.

She had softly gone by the time the nurse got there.

She had softly lived.

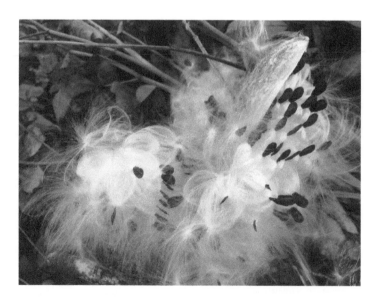

CHANGING

The superintendent held council at his bedside day and night.
With his eyes closed or his eyes open.
His words were perfectly crafted in content and tone:

"The import of what you are saying is of value.
I would like some time to weigh the implications of what you are introducing."

That I couldn't see anyone in the room,
that he had a terminal diagnosis and had come to the inpatient respite house to
die, appeared on the outside irrelevant to him.
He had not stepped down from his position
of political as well as patriarchal power,
what with his deteriorating body and prognosis.
Maybe he hadn't stepped down.
Only a few weeks ago he was still acting as head of the family.

When the grown and educated sons visited,
their father's mind was in a reality we couldn't reach,
his body was incapacitated to stand up on his own,
control his elimination, or swallow food.
The sons whispered in front of their father,
and asked him if he needed anything.

Weeks went by.
Every night the superintendent and father held his captive audience.
As in the day, I was told.
He did not talk to the staff around him. I don't know if he spoke to his sons.
Only to his supervisees with an unbroken constancy, soft and non-aggressive.

I looked for cracks of emotion or a different presence
that might be exposed to make him more accessible to what was ahead of him,
in case he needed a different approach in our job to support him.
I never saw it, nor did it seem he ever saw me or anyone else whom I could see.

One night I came in and he had died.
There was nothing of great incident in the report of the passing.

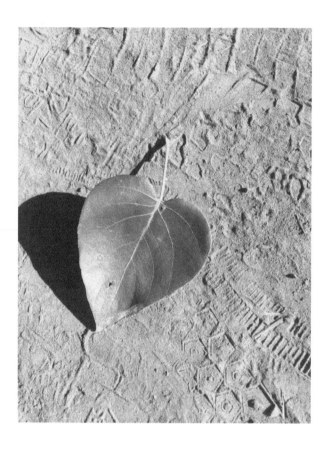

EXCITEAPPOINTMENT

Twitterpated
Then deflated
Drank that coffee
Bladder's aggravated
Mind's all abuzz
As motion slows
Head's apressure cuz
Jitter grows
Can't go down
Same ol' path
Pull that frown
And do the math
It doesn't add
It just subtracts
Not feelin' mad
More like lax
Head's windin' tight
Body goin' under
Tryin' fight or flight
Parts all asunder
Hell's just heaven, in a daze
Twitterflated feeling, is just a phase

~ Troy Maddux, LMT

LOVING A SPANISH PRINCESS

She looked like a Spanish dancer lying in bed
while she had invisible metastasized cancer spread throughout her body.

She was a Spanish dancer.

She was almost always happy. I thought habitually so.
Hand crafts were spread around her as she kept her life going,
almost as if life hadn't transitioned, dying in bed.

As her dexterity was lost, and the focus and distraction of the crafts
could not be held, the openness of the unknown came to question her,
as it does usually.

Sometimes it haunted her. Sometimes it just questioned.
She talked and cried for long hours with her husband in quiet tones.
Long talks that held the silence — talks to which we were not privy.

"She's my babe," he said when I met them both. He looked especially young.
*"When I met her, my friends asked me if it was going to be okay that she is older
than me. Look at her. She's more my babe than ever. I never lost my hots for her."*
He started to cry.

*"When I went to her parents to ask for her hand, I said right off:
'We're great in bed together.'
I wanted to settle that in their minds once and for all."*

It took a while before I noticed that her husband was confined to a wheelchair.

In time he started to get tired living at the Respite House with his Babe,
while not able to take care of his own needs.
We could see him wearing down.
We asked him if he could go home for a night and recoup.

"I made a promise to her when she came here. I am going to keep it.
I told her that I would be with her and not leave her alone at night."

He did as he had promised.

On the final night when she lay in the bed
with her skin tight against her cheeks,
the way the skin falls without wrinkles after we die,
she looking fulfilled and absent at the same time,
he was crumbled over in the chair.

Unable to imagine all the moments of life filled without her.

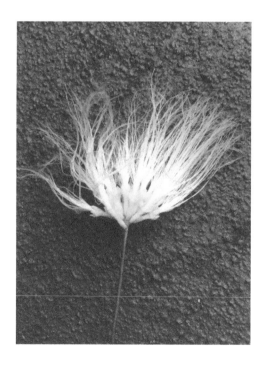

THE VERDICT

One word I thought I would never hear,
One word that may be meant for others but not for me.
One word that resonates and penetrates so deeply
and has no remorse for the arteries it severs in its way.
One word that can never be taken back or ever be forgotten,
One word that does not discriminate,
One word that robs people of their lives.
The verdict is in - you have CANCER

How easy it was for that one word
to slip out of the mouth that told me,
as if it meant nothing.
How difficult it was for my ears to absorb
while I was sitting there all alone.
My head spinning out of control.

It can't be true
It must be wrong
I can't breathe
I can't think
And now I am forced
to make immediate decisions
when that one word
hasn't even had time to fully sink in.

How long do I have?
What will happen to my kids?
Will I die in excruciating pain?
Please!
God!
No!
Wake me up from this nightmare!

I keep hearing people tell me this is your journey,
Journey my ass.
A journey is traveling around the world
or turning over a new leaf.
This isn't a journey at all,
This is a train wreck,
A train that I can't jump off of.
This is a nightmare,
A nightmare I can't wake up from.

With every new change in my body,
Like a verdict returned guilty
to the innocently accused,
I am forever haunted.
This is my new life
A life I didn't choose
Fuck You Cancer!!!

~ Mary Ellis, RN

DON'T WAIT

"S.O.G. for 'Stupid Old Guy', was my nickname." The other carpenters who worked with him had similar nicknames.

"I miss working. I know some people wait for days off of work, but I miss the guys. We worked hard, but we put a lot of houses together. I liked to drive around and see what we had done. We did some great places."

When I walked in on another night with his midnight morphine, and called him by his nickname, he looked surprised at first, and then smiled, *"You remembered."*

Before I had time to say anything, he lamented, *"If there is anything you want to do, don't wait."*

He was 58.

"I had plans. I had started making fly hooks. My shop was all set up. It took a long time to put together everything I needed. They were perfect. And they worked. The guys have to take over my stuff now. Maybe someone else will do it."

The night was quiet. No call-bells were ringing. I sat at the edge of the bed and listened to the night's space.

"There are a lot of places I wanted to see. There is a waterfall just off our ride home. It was one I particularly wanted to see. It was late one day when we thought of stopping. I thought we would get another chance. I didn't."

I wished his body could still tolerate a visit to the waterfall. We pondered it. He saw it as a past opportunity when he could hang with the boys.

At first when he arrived at the inpatient hospice house, he kept his door closed all the time. Actually, that never changed. But what did change was that he kept it closed for quiet — not to keep people away. He talked more, he cried more, he teased more, he changed. He changed from wanting to keep to himself for weeks and weeks, to craving company and telling the aides that he loved them.

"She's great," he said about a boisterous aide who did everything big. Her face was very dark in skin color and she had learned how to keep people from pushing her around. When she walked into the room with her big movements and gruff hello, he would smile hugely with the love of gratitude.

It was she, and those who worked with her, who tended to every detail that his incapacitated body could no longer do for itself, and for which he was now dependent on others. His beard looked like he had just come from the barber. His room smelled good. Everything he needed was where he needed it in reach, when he needed it.

His pain took longer to get under control than we are happy to admit. He had the kind of pain that is the hardest: Equally wedded to the body as to the mind and spirit and emotions.

And it was monstrous pain.

The chaos of the changing over of nurse managers let more days slip through than my conscience can bear when I look back. It took stronger psych medications than what we started, to attack the bone pain plus the mental agony plus the memory pain. Memory pain is pain that is worse every time it happens because it triggers your memory from all the intolerable pain you have had up to then.

It is also true, as my dearest colleague reminded me, when I was verbalizing my agony over this, that he had refused a pain medication infusion pump for weeks, along with refusing other treatments,when he still thought personal control was the key to relief.

He let go of pieces of his control little by little. And we got our act together.

Still he fought. He didn't want to die. He would get angry. Scared. He had profound, tearful conversations with his wife. They weren't easy. He told her how he felt. She cried too. He yelled at us sometimes. He cried easily and often.

Finding Justice in the shortness of his life, when he thought he would and should have so many more years, never came.

His last night was after walking and talking the day before. He had battled; then just let go. He blew out the candle. With his wife in the room.

He wasn't either stupid or old, and his nickname paraded him.

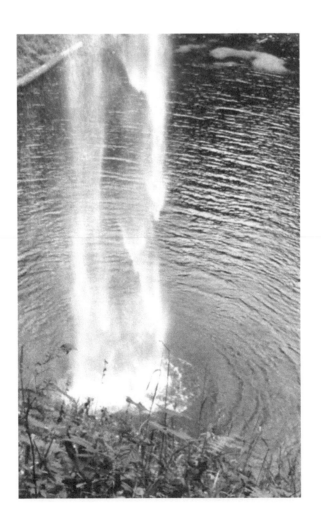

CRYING

Spent so many years of crying
In hurt and loss and shame,
Now it seems that I'm not trying
It seems I'm not the same.
I'm swimming in a world of grief
From north and south, east and west,
I look and see the fallen leaf
Multicolored death vest.
Somehow prettier than the green
Though photosynthesizing no more,
What I hold is what I've seen
The other stuff I store.
I don't cry now when I'm low
And it makes me wonder why,
Cry I will in a movie show
When fictional characters die.
Doesn't make sense when I logic it out
It must not be this way.

~ Troy Maddux, LMT

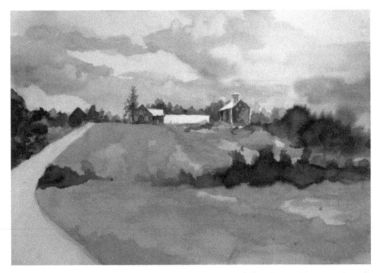

© Ink by Anya Katrina Smith

THE CLOSING SIGNATURE

Her husband built her a mansion that housed her needs in grandeur. She had severe physical limitations long before now. It was as they wanted it at home: The jacuzzi under a picture window looking out at Mount Mansfield… I had images in my mind from what I heard. She was young and she was to die at home. Everything had been planned and arranged. All attended to.

Except that at home she couldn't get a handle on the pain. They fought tenaciously. The Home Health nurses got called in more and more frequently. Then she needed round-the-clock care, and still the pain was out of control. That's when we met her and her husband who did not leave her side.

"She's here just to get her pain under control. Then she is going back home to die."

That was the report of their intention. We were on it. She didn't connect with us the way some other residents did. Her connection was with her husband and her home. He spoke for her.

Every day we got closer to meeting her body in the way it needed for relief. But it took a few days before the complex breakthrough pain was under control and before she maintained some levelness and predictability in her relief. The problem was that she arrived looking already like she was about to die.

We didn't have time.

There was almost nothing left covering her skeleton. When she got up to the bedside commode, (she insisted that she could still do it and would not hear otherwise). She would faint each time. And she would have it no other way. Almost all she would say is, *"When am I going home?"*

She looked like someone who would no longer be able to speak. Then all she could say was, *"Home?"*

Her son had died very young. She had told her husband that on the way home she wanted to stop at her son's grave-site.

It seemed inconceivable.

On the final day, I left work late because she was in crisis. Crisis only because death was close and she was not home. She had passed out again. She had stopped breathing. She had emptied her GI tract like people do sometimes after they die. Her skin was mottled as happens when the blood goes to the vital organs, away from the extremities, and the red blood cells break down under the skin surface. Her complexion was ashen. Her skin cold. It seemed as if she had died. Most of the physical signs of death were there.

Except that her breath came back. Her erratic racing thready heartbeat that was so faint it could almost not be palpated, kept on.

At 10:00 am the ambulance was to come to take her back home. At 8:30 am when I left, I couldn't imagine her making it another hour, much less making a stressful trip. I got the update when I went back to work the next night:

She had got into the ambulance, the ambulance had stopped at the cemetery on the way home. They had gotten her in her own bed. I was told she smiled and looked up at the mountain through the skylight above her bed. Her family was with her. At 1 pm she died:

Where and when she said she would. No sooner, No later, Nowhere but home. She called it. Against all odds. Against death itself… Or with death.

The ambulance company refused any pay.

I began to get it, with her, how much more we get to ask for than we think. Even in the face of the uncontrollable. Where we get our final signature.

MAKE SURE THEY KNOW

"I was just thinking about you," she said as I walked into the room. It was time for her daily 6 am enema. Partial bowel obstruction. Secondary to colon cancer.

Her quiet, pensive mode was notable. She was a hospice nurse by profession. She seemed especially calm. The previous day she said with defiance that she was done with them (the enemas). Until she followed through in her head the consequences of declining it — and ended up with, *"Well, if you put it that way!"*

"I was thinking about how kind you are to me," she said, finishing her welcoming statement. Two nights ago she had said, *"I get so spoiled here, I'm going to wish to not die."* We laughed at that. It felt good to laugh heartily. When she could breathe again, she said, *"How did I come up with that?"*

After coffee, I said to her, "You are a brave woman." *"I hope so,"* she said. The sun was coming out. We were in no hurry. Life is too short, I reminded myself, to be in a hurry too often.

"My legs are pretty funny looking. And look at this," she said, patting her distended abdomen that sounded like a drum. "Every day your body is less important," I contributed, being more preachy than was helpful, as she lay making skin-and-bones and fluid and gas, a live thing.

"I know that," she said, *"But I like to see it as funny too. I want my family to see that side as well. My toes look like little pillows. It would be even funnier if my breasts got puffed up. They look like fried eggs. JesusMaryandJoseph. Now that's pretty funny!"*

She talked with a mixture of humor and womanly loss. *"My sister complains about having too much. She says they flop over when she turns. I feel sooo bad for her. Ugh!"*

She reminded me to laugh even in hard things. Maybe especially through the hard stuff. When we were quiet again; I asked, "Are you scared of dying?" I was pretty sure I knew her answer.

"No," she said simply — without needing to contemplate. "*I want to be an example for my grandchildren… especially after the way my husband died.*"

A long time ago her husband took an over-dose of medication when he heard he had early Parkinson's, and died in the hospital three weeks later.

Mopsie (as she likes to be called after her grandson started calling her that) spoke easily about her deceased husband, and brought him into her life at the Respite House in big and small ways.

"*He would have liked this glass for his scotch,*" she had said before she fell asleep last night. "*The ridges make it less slippery,*" she noted, giving careful attention to the design and texture of the water glass that was exuding condensation with clear drips onto her sheet, as she held it in her hand.

"Do you have any requests of me as you go through this?" I asked her. This she did contemplate for a long time. She finally said, with a lot of pauses and re-starts, "*Well, if I do things or act in ways that are not in the spirit we are talking about… if I get mean, or… say things that… hurt anyone, will you remind me what I told you about wanting to do this differently? Will you remind me that I don't want to do it that way, and help bring me back?*"

Now it was turn for me to ponder. I want to see all behavior as a clue into someone's inner turmoil or peace, and in a professional environment, meeting up with that, versus correcting or reminding, or even focusing on different behavior. But she was asking about her presentation while communicating with her family.

Maybe it is not so different than what I had asked of my midwife at the birth of my first daughter. "Remind me through each contraction that it's my baby." That is what had gotten me through my first natural birthing in joy.

"Well, let's talk this out," I said — now me fumbling for words. "I am used to doing the opposite. Your mental status could change. You could do and say things that are not truly you; we've been there before together. I take my job as accepting behaviors, and seeing them as a gift for companioning. In knowing you, whatever you do and have done, I don't and wouldn't see it as mean. Even if you started yelling at me, even if you swung out at me.

"But, yes, I will do what I can to help you bring your spirit to the forefront. Also, I accept your actions in their variety. Especially when you would be having a hard time. I would know and reflect back to you the person I know you are."

She looked at me.

"That might help you be less hard on yourself. You have had a lot to go through. Maybe what I can do is remind your daughter of these things if you go through hard times like that and she gets confused."

She looked out the window with a clarity and serenity that was tangible. *"Maybe I can tell her that myself,"* she said. *"Yes, I will talk to her."*

The sun was a bit higher. The flowers in the gardens drank in the morning light. She seemed to be talking to herself. *"I am going to tell them how much I love them, how very much I love them all. I am going to make sure they know that."*

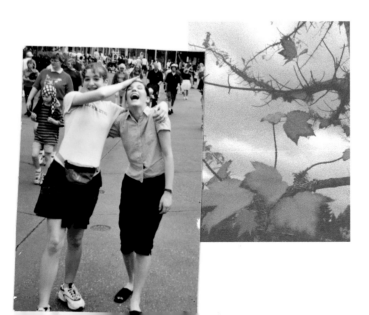

THE BIRD NEST

When I hear the scratching of the bush on the window screen, when the birds come to it each spring, I remember the young man in his 50s who had been in a wheelchair since he was nineteen or so, from a car accident. Frank was his name.

What kind of cancer grew in later years, now is forgotten to me. It was not that, but a cavernous pressure ulcer that he could not feel (with his paraplegia from his accident) that caused sepsis in the end, and took his life.

I actually rarely saw that, because the dressing change was done on the day shift, and he took care of most other things himself. Like the tube he stuck into his abdomen to release urine. The nursing aides saw more of that than I did, even at night, when they helped him with his personal care. I rarely even saw his thin legs at night under the blankets. His upper body was built-up from an active life, exercise, and wheelchair-propelling.

It was many years ago, but my memory of him feels like yesterday's. He had an energetic sense about him. The room he lived in remains his in my consciousness. He looked a lot like Kenny Rogers. He loved the sun. His skin around his neatly trimmed red beard was leathery thick and dark — the orange-brown that farmers get from the fields. Or like the skin of the Indians in the high altitude of *La Sierra Madre* in Mexico.

The wrinkles around his eyes were cheerful wrinkles from a mischievous grinning face that was angry as often as it was teasing.

His father's portrait, placed carefully where he could see it from his bed, was an austere black-and-white photo of a man with a hat and gun who met hardship, the son said, without stepping back. To me the dad looked like he stood feeling alone — if he had thought about that, which he most likely didn't. Can you feel alone if you don't think about it and are not conscious of it?

I doubt the dad found the time, energy, or space between drinks to contemplate his existence and its effect on people like himself or his son. But who knows.

Clearly his son wanted to be like him. And at the same time the son was proud he wasn't like his dad. The son was soft inside and didn't keep it too far hidden to discover. He tried very hard to present himself like his dad on the outside; but he couldn't. He cared too much about both himself as well as those around him.

The first day I met him he chastised me for something I couldn't understand being my responsibility. It was a long time ago now. I thought I was going to connect with him right away and he sent me out of his room. Whatever he would berate or try to battle with, seems inconsequential in retrospect. Even at the time it felt less than important than his clear desire and simultaneous fear to connect.

He was a remarkably light sleeper. No matter how quietly I snuck into his room, even with my practiced light step for night checks, he would instantly open his eyes. I noted it out loud. *"I learned that young. I never knew when my dad would be coming in."* [To beat him.] The hard life was matter-of-fact to Frank. His nightmares, nervousness, and mistrust of people was not. His symptom-management was as complex as his persona. It was hard work — for everyone, him included. For him most of all. "What is the best thing that has happened to you in your life?" I asked him once.

"My accident," he said, stopping in his track and thinking. I asked him why. There was clarity in his voice: *"For one, if I had not had my accident I wouldn't be here today. And that's for sure. I was headed down a dangerous path. The law and me did not see things eye to eye. I wasn't stupid enough to get caught. My dad and I never got caught. But I would be dead today if I had not gotten off that path."* He looked out the window. *"In those days I would never have done what I do now: I wouldn't want the guys to know, but I watch those baby birds in the bush. I can quiet myself now in ways I didn't know existed. It's something I didn't know anything about before."*

In the breeze the bush made its presence known against the window screen.

The sun was almost up. The birds back and forth to the nest were hidden from the outside, but could be seen from inside the window. They reflected a focused busyness as a stark contrast to their friend in the bed. Later in the day this complex man would go outside in the sun, sitting for hours on his wheelchair, the sun beating on his body. His body understood the outdoors and the outdoors came to understand the man at one with simple things.

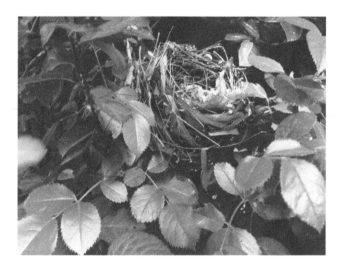

1957

She was a hospice nurse (the same patient I told you about earlier). Cancer and heart disease brought her to the respite house to die. This is what she told me of now dated hospice work in 1957:

"It makes me sick when I think of it. They used to pull their hair out in pain. Literally. A guy who had pancreatic cancer pulled it out in chunks at a time. He was just one. The doctors wouldn't prescribe enough medication. They were afraid of 'hastening death' and afraid of addiction. It was 1957 when I graduated from nursing school.

The man with dermal cancer didn't have half his face. It was hard to feed him. The food would pour out. The smell was so bad, no one would stop to talk. We just did the treatments as fast as we could and got out of there. His family couldn't handle visiting him.

I decided to take him on. I tried putting Vicks under my nose. It distracted the smell. I talked with him. We laughed.

I asked him how long since his windows had been washed. I cleaned them and made a scene of it. I danced and made a fool of myself. Anything as an excuse to show him I liked being with him.

My colleagues said they were worried about me. I started losing weight. I couldn't get rid of that smell, even when I wasn't in his room. I lost my appetite."

"Did you use Flagyl?" I asked impulsively. (Crushing Flagyl onto an open necrotic wound, helps.) "I know our latest aromatherapy distributors are pretty newly developed." I knew immediately I was off in my comments. And we both knew that even these were at best partially effective interventions of something that had only one remedy: Being connected to the human behind the wounds and smell.

"No," she continued. "*I asked my supervisor if I could talk to his wife about going to see him,*" she continued. My supervisor said that if it went badly, she would back me. I talked to the wife. She loved him. She said that when she went in and tried to stay, she would dry-heave. She tried the Vicks. It helped…"

There was a long pause.

"*It's hard to think that I'm dying,*" the hospice nurse patient went on. "*I'm not getting my gallbladder removed. I'm not going in for radiation. I came here to die. I can't get my head around it.*"

"I can't either," I said. "It seems elusive. No one gets it. It is rather bigger than us, I think." We looked out the window together on a beautiful fresh summer morning. A rabbit jumped across the grass, making the half cement one (with its butt sticking up out of the ground) look sort of funny and out-of-place. At least the live rabbit was not the one looking out-of-place.

"You know," I said, "thinking of dying feels like the ultimate loss of control. 'Cause we can't get out of it, any of us. But you know what is amazing?" She looked at me. "People here seem to find a way to orchestrate their death. Like who is with them when they die, the specific timing of it… it's hard to explain. They make arrangements with people we can't see or hear.

It's like their final earthly signature. I don't know how they do it, but they do." We looked at each other for a while.

"*I'm starving,*" she said. "*I'm sick of this diet the doctor put me on. She better know what she is doing because I'm damn sick of this soft food stuff.*" (She had just gotten past a bowel obstruction and had graduated from a liquid to a soft foods diet.)

"How about some tapioca to start?" I offered. "There is a fresh batch. You can eat all you want to, and after tonight you can eat whatever you want." Tomorrow would be the first day she was going to try to eat more solid foods.

"I'm sick of everything on that list," she said. "Tapioca sounds good, though."

She smiled when I came back, and fell asleep after her bowl of tapioca.

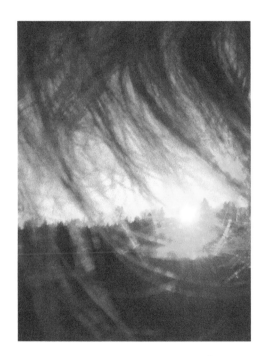

EXCEPT FOR SITT'N STILL

I thought she couldn't get up on her own: Parkinsons.

Difficulty with initiating movement.

She had the strength, but getting her to use it was the challenge:

Getting her out of the chair, up in the morning, dressed… took her time.

That said, one afternoon, when a toddler was playing before her armchair,

and the toddler then stood up and was about to fall over,

Sara was in time to catch him in seconds.

We all turned around. There was silence in the room.

There she stood, no one near her but the child.

She had been in the recliner seconds before.

"X 1-2 assist for transfers / fall risk" – is what the nursing notes said.

For any other move, I blocked out time for her, because that is what it took:

quite a bit of time to get her from sitting to standing

and then pivoting into the wheelchair.

Maybe she could take a few steps, but no more than that,

and all with a significant amount of assistance.

Not on this occasion.

I guess once a mom always a mom.

She was an English teacher too.

Quips and poems danced with facile presence on her tongue.

Our English was corrected in our own home.

I guess once a teacher, always a teacher.

We didn't get away with much under her tutelage.

I have a binder of her quips

(that I recorded and gave to the family at the time of her death):

Her hair was a '*don't*' — more than a '*hair do*'.
She was certain it was only the paper company that was benefiting
from the incontinence briefs.
"*I'll be suing you,*"
is what I got for a goodnight in answer to my, 'I'll be seeing you'.

She died with her beloved daughter Suzanne squeezed into the adjustable bed,
lying by her side in her arms, at the crescendo of Amazing Grace.

Until we get double adjustable beds as an option
with the durable medical suppliers, we are at a deficit.
Renting two adjustable beds to be placed side-by-side is the interim option
for family and partners, but hospice does not yet cover two per patient.
It is not just couples who scrunch themselves next to their dying partners,
ignoring the discomfort of the narrow beds we rent.

Sara was the first person I nursed in death at our family residential care home
where we chose to work so we could be with our children while they grew up,
and they could learn from the work.

My now ex-husband ran the business-side of it with his expertise and diligence,
along with many hours of other work outside of the home.
I did the housework with the patients, our family, and our loved ones —
the cooking, the cleaning, the extensive gardening, the caregiving.
We had some expert nurse aide help, and respite help too
to try to get away once a month. That was great when it worked.
We worked hard around-the-clock
in ways we could never sustain today at an older age.
I remember I did not sleep much. (Sometimes that is still true, I guess.)
My Ex and I were good counterparts in business for what we named,
Silver Wings Residential Care.

Anya, our youngest, was the perfect unifier for all ages
of both people and pets.
For the older daughter, it was a hard adjustment, and not a welcome one.

For the very oldest of my ex-husband's, she had already moved out of home,
and she experienced it from a distance.
For the adopted daughter, it made a new life for her possible,
being the one foster child we adopted.
For our 'borrowed daughter', as we called her, of dear family friends,
it gave a period of reprieve and healing at a time in her life that she needed it,
and that we needed her.
For Sara, for them, and for the many pets, it was home.

When it was time to bury Sara,
our then 5-year-old daughter skipped around the open grave
as the casket went down.
"I am glad I shared my cat with her," Anya said,
as the adults cried, overwhelmed with the cloud of loss.
Sara thought Anya's cat was her own, not Anya's,
and it was one of Anya's first experiences of letting perceived ownership go
for camaraderie and someone else's happiness,
and the truth that we are but stewards, not owners.

To date Anya sits down with people of any age as if they were peers.
She got practiced at it.
Along then with her rabbits and birds and cats and dog and rats and hamsters
for pets, and along with her love for the flowers,
which she was the first to catch the latest bloom.
All of that today remains close to her heart and life.
To date Samantha, the adopted daughter, is a Nurse Aide,
in the spirit of the home in which she grew up.

Sara asked to be buried in a field there,
thinking she was back in Pennsylvania where she grew up.
In later years, when I went to Sara's grave-site,
I could feel the instant peace and companionship that she gave me
when we lived and shared.
It was one of my favorite spots,
near a child swing and an adult swing, hung from the ancient apple trees.

Our neighbor carried a huge rock to the gravesite with his bull-dozer.
There, in my heart, lay her morning poem:

I wisht I was a little rock
a- sittn' on a hill.
A doin' nothin' all day long, but just a sittin' still.
I wouldn't eat, I wouldn't sleep,
I wouldn't even wash.
I'd sit and sit a thousand years,
And rest myself by Gosh!

~ Anonymous

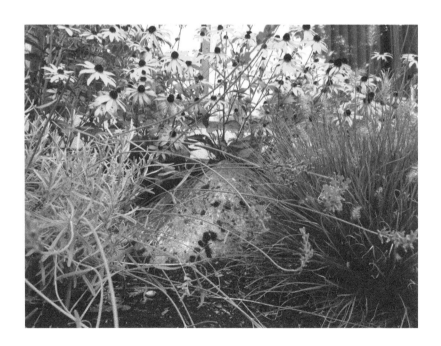

ENERGY

Energy; sounds like the letters NRG, which in my case will probably stand for 'Not Really Gonna' as in not really gonna do it. But then here I am doing just what I said that I was not really gonna do. So in the words of Buckaroo Bonzai, "no matter where you go, there you are." Genius. Which is a word that sounds like Jenie and Us, like maybe we all have magic in us. Wouldn't that be great if we were all magical and all capable of something so much greater than we have ever seen. Wouldn't it be great if we could take something mundane and make it sublime, take something ridiculous and make it heavenly? Heaven, that's a concept: a place of all that good that goes on forever and ever, something that humankind has aspired to for millenia and yet what do we consume? In the words and in the images and in the flickering pictures we look for pain and suffering and things that are hard and those that are at odds. Such a contrast, such a paradox to fill our lives with the opposite of what we say we want. But then maybe that is the human condition to hold dissimilar and even opposing forces in the same space to see how they dance, to see what they will create.

~ Troy Maddux, LMT

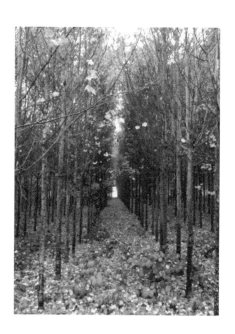

PRETTY PEOPLE

Everyone likes pretty people. We notice them in a crowd, we steal glances at them across a room, we want to go and talk to them and listen to these pretty people talking to us. It is exciting somehow. Maybe it is just our genes calling out to motivate us to find the fittest and the ones that look the best have the healthiest children.

It makes me wonder maybe these aren't the best people to talk to. Maybe our lives are woven from and interwoven with stories and stories that hook us and create stronger bonds with others in our community. Maybe all the adulation and attention tends to turn the stories of pretty people toward themselves, and how people fawn over them and those stories, doesn't interest the listener and doesn't burn a groove in the brain or the heart but burns away like a morning mist; magical for a moment then dissipating in the bright sunshine.

Give me stories of the maimed and misshapen, the stories of the pained and the broken, the stories of the cast-off and neglected. Stories of struggles and victories over them, maybe only partial victories or temporary, but the taste on the tongue and the tingle in the toes of it stays with them and carries them forward. Forward with hope of a better world. A world with more hope and less despair and more connection and less isolation and more laughter, fewer tears, more closeness and less neglect. Where stories of love weave all together, the pretty people and the plain.

~ Troy Maddux, LMT

FRIENDS AND FAMILY

When I went to visit Paula in her home,
she sat on her couch with her cat resting next to her.
I was visiting her the night before my wedding to my tango partner.
She said she wanted to go to the wedding.
Her eyes dropped to half-mast during most of the short visit.
She was quick to smile, slow to move.

"I can do things if I move very slowly," she told me that night.
"Even a bike ride," she said.

She was dying.
In another month she would be at her last days,
very soon after she was diagnosed.
Very soon after, I remember her stretching on the tango room floor,
looking like a picture of beauty and health.

As a hospice nurse I don't usually meet patients in their physical prime.
Paula, I did know with her physical power.
Tonight, the night before my wedding, that was her prime too.

She tangoed slowly.
It was hard to get used to the difference
of the calculated energy of every move,
with her misted sight that seemed to see beyond the moment.
We knew her as vivacious, and verbally outspoken, in the present.

Yet her centeredness in what is lasting was palpable
in those two days that I saw her.
There was no time or strength for anything but the forever:

Her love with her family and friends.

Michael writing about Paula:

WILLFULNESS

For reasons that are a whole other story, and against all common sense and past history, I decided to become a tango dancer. The initial angst and misery — which lasted almost a year — were intense enough so all I could focus on was watching my feet plod forward, trying to not step on my kind partners who were mostly a blur. Eventually I began to actually become aware of some of the dancers as distinct humans and not just bodies I was trying to not harm too much.

Paula was one of the first because she was just so warm, open, supportive and excited to be dancing. She reminded me of a popular book from our mutual college years titled, 'Be Here Now!' I don't know if she ever read it — it was by Baba Ram Dass… whose name says it all, I guess — but she sure seemed to live it.

As time went on I began to kind of actually learn to dance and, once again, one of the first people that it was easy with was Paula. She never was judgmental or frustrated with mistakes and, increasingly, we were really dancing and flowing and it was great.

But here is the core of Paula: She could not be contained! Her energy kept spiraling up. We would be totally in sync but then, quite suddenly, she would accelerate and strange things would happen; she would start inventing new things far beyond my skill level and things would collapse into giggles and chaos. Then she would look me in the eye, laugh and say, "Oops, I'm being willful." and we would start again. As I improved I learned to respond without collapse; I'd reign us in and we'd keep going with hardly anybody being aware and I loved to let her loose. But she would lean in and whisper, "I was being willful again!" as we lightly circled the line of dance.

~ Mickey Tango nee' Michael Wisniewski

Scott writing about Paula:

I first met Paula several years ago at an Argentine tango beginners' lesson in Burlington. She was wearing a flower print dress and military boots, she had fire in her eyes and seemed to have arrived prepared for combat. The dance of tango, by its nature, requires a certain strategic aggressiveness on the part of its leaders and, correspondingly, a certain playful submissiveness on the part of its followers. I didn't initially have the impression that Paula was aware of these concepts, and, if she did, she must have had her own notions as to how the dance was to be done, i.e. her way or the highway. Needless to say, I was a bit apprehensive about my prospects of taming her. Happily, however, tango has a way of bringing balance to its participants through assertion, compromise and the reality of biomechanics; and so it was after many lessons, practicas and milongas, I believe Paula and I reached an understanding of sorts as to how to organize our willpower on the dance floor and celebrate together the artful passion of the tango dance. Along the way, I came to know Paula and the delightfully feisty, generous and loving person that she was.

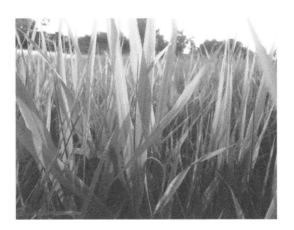

SPEED

Speed is what I was thinking about yesterday or maybe it was slowing down; slowing down and opening up more space to allow things to unfold and unfurl.

If you keep a chrysalis in a small jar the butterfly ends up with twisted and stunted wings. If you try to hurry the process and open the cage then damage occurs.

Slow came up after I held the small of the back for a patient having pain there and how comforting that was, how powerful that was.

Why do I not slow down in every aspect of my life? Open up spaces in my schedule because in the spaces the magic happens. That is where yogis say to be is in the space between the exhale and the inhale.

The place of stillness, the space, the place of magic.

Breathe and slow down, open space and allow the natural unfurling of that which is.

Slow, open, be, breathe, ahhhhhhh.

~ Troy Maddux, LMT

"El Tiempo No Existe, y No Hay Apura."

(Time Doesn't Exist, and There Is No Hurry.)

~ Madrid, Spain Airport Wall

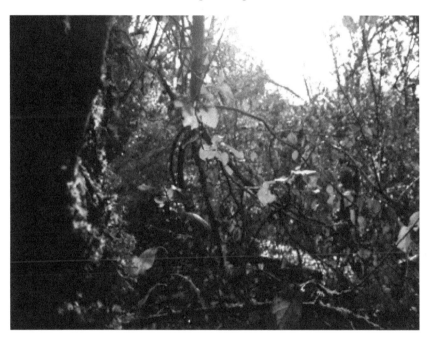

"Nothing is too much trouble when one loves, and there is always time."

~ Abdú'l-Bahá

TAIL OF THE WORLD

"You've got the world by its tail
And it's hanging upside down,"
She said to me
And if she could
She'd do it for me,
Live my life
The way it should be lived,
With eagerness and warmth,
And with abandon.
And she would get it right
My life
I can see it in her eyes
Crying tears of joy for all the love she's known,
The love that still sustains her
Past a reasonable age,
Love already spilling over to another realm.
And if I could
I'd do it for her
Die her death
The way it should be done
With sweet anticipation of
An endless
Calm.
And I would get it right.

~Mary Brutsaert, LCSW

Part Two

THE VALLEY OF LOVE

You are the Boss

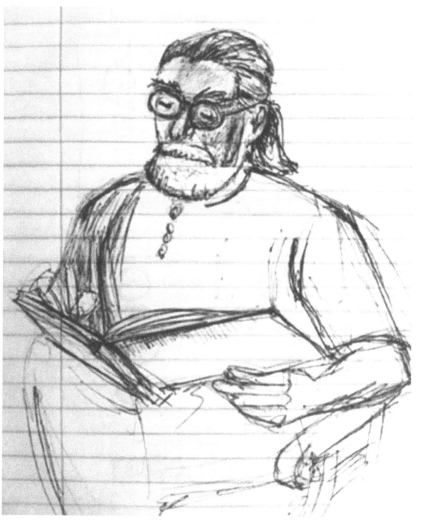

© Courtesy of Mike Lavigne *(Portrait of son at his mother's bedside during her last days.)*

AS IT IS

"You are vertical," I commented in the kitchen
as the 21-year-old Russian woman made herself some breakfast in the kitchen.
She laughed,
being new (though fluent) to the English language and its nuances.
I was at work for a day meeting and usually talked to Yvonne
when she was lying in bed, horizontal, next to her husband every night,
amidst every kind of tube and orifice intrusion on the books, it seemed.

That he was 60-years-old and she 21, he malodorous and she as sweet as youth,
he irritable, she even-tempered,
he ensnared in drain tubes and artificial apparatuses
for administering and eliminating bodily needs,
she seemingly oblivious of that impact on their love.
All seemed, at the time, to bypass Yvonne's consciousness.
She would lie there on her side, in the one spot
where she wouldn't disturb the intruding stuff,
stroking the parts of his skin that she could reach.

Her face expressed intensity, newness, the unknown, fear, affection.
Never distaste.

For him, overshadowing all else, was his adoration of her.
Constant singular focus of his love and infatuation,
outside of his physical misery.
She felt it.
He had been married to someone else most of his life,
and had recently married Yvonne.
He had no desire left in life but to settle his finances
so that they would go to his new wife.
(To the great challenge of his ex-wife who was not going to let go easily.)

It is rare when money is a focus at death.

Maybe even in this case it was not really the money,

but what the money would do for the woman in his heart

whom he was leaving behind.

Their detailed story is lost in the shuffle of writing,

and my detailed memories lost to time.

What remains is the complete grace of the Russian woman, with what was,

and his devotion.

Later she described it as a world unto itself

where the darkness took a long time to dispel.

Years later I came across her at JC Penney

and I recognized Yvonne as the cashier.

We were delighted to see each other.

She was, yes, vertical, smiling and not sleep-deprived.

She was employed after being taken care of by her husband before he died.

She had a young sweet Russian boyfriend her age

who did not have any tubes and decaying body smells.

Her face expressed intensity, newness, the unknown, affection.

Relaxed, confident, young, easy.

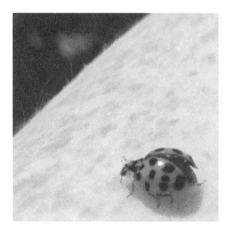

LAUGHING OUT LOUD

They stood there
Three kids
Looking at their dead mother
And they laughed
Out loud together.
They laughed about the
Awfulness of it all
Caring for their mother
All these months,
Watching her descend further and further into
Confusion and forgetfulness;
Seeing her give up her English properness and
Allow others to wash her and change her;
Hearing her say, near the end,
This is worse than the war -
The London bombings she had survived in WWII.
They laughed
Remembering her proclaim
How she had finally figured it out,
The only explanation her failing brain could come up with
As to why this being alive business kept on going
Long past any reasonable point:
"You all hate me!"
They laughed
For several seconds
Connected by their
Mother's body
Still warm.

They laughed about what they had endured together
What they had survived together.
They laughed to find out
There is life
Even after this.

~ Mary Brutsaert, LCSW

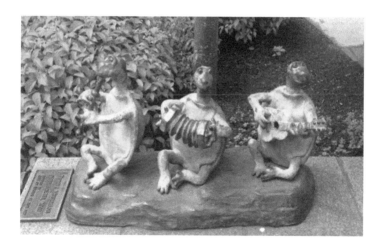

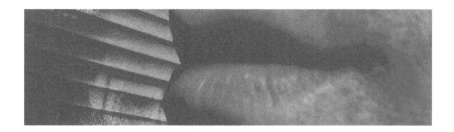

THE YOUNG MUSLIM

He was albino and very young. It was a demanding night for the nurses, and the evening nurse forgot to give me an overview of the new patient before I walked into his room to see huge black cancer growths the size of grapefruits, growing from the side of his face. Despite being practiced at seeing people as people, past their disrupted bodies, it would have helped if I hadn't needed a second or two to evaluate what I was seeing, before showing that I understood he was more than the atrocity of his tumors.

He was in his twenties. Later we found out he might have been younger than we already thought he was young, but no one had tracked his birthday. Muhammad was his guide. His Faith was such that no human powers, no physical bodily power, no mammoth gnarling growths that stared back at him in the mirror, daunted his spirit or broke his seriousness of focus, most of the time. At first I couldn't remember a smile, much less a laugh from him, but I may have missed them, being it was nighttime. Once he got used to us, and us to him, a naturalness of comfort, and even a quiet humor evolved.

No collapsing of spirit… Except on the one night. Surely other times he struggled to keep his faith. We all do. But I rarely saw it. He prayed throughout the day, as dictated by the Islamic religion. He said that Muhammad called the shots, not the doctors, nor anyone else. He said he would live when Muhammad called it, and would die when Muhammad called it. Not I, not the doctor, nor anyone else, had the answers.

He was getting radiation for comfort to reduce his tumors. It would not take away the cancer, the doctors said, because there was too much of the disease. The intent was to help manage the size of the growths. He was a hospice patient, not a palliative patient. That means his doctor assessed him to have six months or less to live, supposing the disease progressed on its projected course. That meant that the most expert treatments no longer had the expectation of curing. He played the piano in the daytime. It was elementary, but he said he wanted to learn. He got on a bike and circled the parking lot, round and round and round. He loved the bicycle. He was not allowed off the premises for fear of medical needs coming up while he was out.

He was deeply contemplative at night, and deeply pensive. He asked for bananas throughout his wakeful hours, and fruit. We ordered extra bananas to stock just for him. He spent much of the dark hours in prayer. At first he spoke to no one except as obliged; he seemed in his own world. Then in the daytime it was said he became playful and engaging as he got used to people, and worked on his broken English, of which he spoke almost none when he arrived.

One night I suddenly realized that his tumors were disappearing. I had not focused on them until it was mentioned in a care meeting. He was clearly (of course) elated at the change. He said he wanted to see the doctor about it. The doctor came to see him the next day, and said that it was not the cancer healing. She said it was just the radiation diminishing the tumors.

That is the night that his spirit crashed. He had thought Muhammad was answering his prayers. Now the doctor was telling him that he was not better. He felt better. He was deeply dejected. He was quiet for long dark hours.

Then he sat up straight from his lying position, crossed his legs, and said, with a mixture of resolution and anger, that no one, not doctors, not any human of any position or power or education, knew his future. That is when he said to me with complete clarity and conviction that if Muhammad wanted him to die young, that he would die young. If Muhammad wanted him to live longer, then he would live longer.

I asked for a higher protein diet in the daytime for his healing. An evening nurse thought of that. The answer from the doctor was to not get his hopes up. She said it didn't matter what he ate because his cancer was not curable.

His tumors disappeared anyway. So did he from the inpatient hospice house. He moved from hospice to palliative care.

Months went by.

I asked about him a year later from our new nurse manager who had taken to him and had followed his doings. She said that he had his own apartment, that she had seen him walking in town. With his head held high, wearing a hat, and that he paraded an extra large and especially shiny belt buckle.

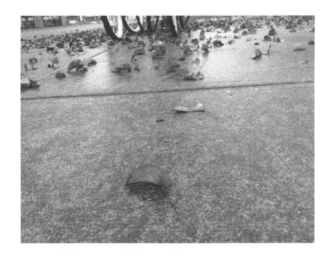

THE CLOSING OF TWO LIVES

Life ebbs and flows.

I went to Boston to visit my first-born daughter. We each bought a new styling hat to walk the streets. In our new look we engaged with the subway young men searching their mark and dance. Probably not so different than Kate's and my donning our new hats. A young man took center stage, standing on his head as the subway moved. He then commenced a monologue that in words offended, but in spirit smelled like an effort at engagement in a Bostonian culture of social distance.

My daughter and I started the day glum in a cold city, and ended the day holding hands, laughing, light, together.

I remember taking a breath around 7 pm and thinking of Diane at the Respite House. I marked the time; wondering if it was significant back in Diane's world. I found out when I got back to Vermont that Diane had died at 7:10 pm. The same time I had felt a flush of her consciousness. I thought she had come to say good-bye to me when I could not be there for her.

When I saw her paperwork outside of the 'Current Patients' binder, I looked up on the board to see her name erased. I turned off the tears that wanted to come, and wore instead my more professional demeanor. Not that crying at work is inappropriate. But it was the start of a new shift and I had a lot that needed tending.

Plus I knew Diane wasn't gone. Still, I missed her already. I asked descriptive questions: She had been peaceful, I was told, her son had been with her. It was a quiet, non-dramatic death.

Like her.

Before I could reflect much more, the word was that Alan in Giraffe Room was in acute respiratory distress and agitation. Another night to hit the floor on-mark.

Alan, a husband and father, was in the Giraffe Room. He was mostly non-responsive throughout the day and night, and then all of a sudden he would talk to you, answer questions, and be 'all there'. Until he wasn't again. He had a gentleness about him that was also unexpected because he seemed like the kind of guy who was going to bark at you or say rationally incongruent things in a seemingly altered state of mind. And then, instead, he would give you eye-contact and have clear wants and refusals. No explanations. Just on occasion a quiet clarity of mind and speech.

Dawn, his wife, and Barbara, his daughter, were visiting him every day, spending most of every day with him.

Then, on the same day that my youngest, almost-18-year-old daughter, skidded out of control over the ice on our dirt road driving home from school, Barbara and Dawn left VRH to go home, and lost control on another icy road. They hit a tree. The car was destroyed. So was Dawn's body. The daughter, Barbara, was practically untouched. Dawn did not have on a seat belt. The side air bags reportedly exploded out, protecting Barbara from hitting her head on the window. She has but a slight bruise on her hip at the site of the seatbelt buckle. Dawn was thrown about the car. The grandson was driving behind them and watched it happen. Dawn's back reportedly broke in 3 places. Also broken were her hip, clavicle, several ribs… A collapsed lung… She was in Intensive Care.

That day no one came to visit Alan. He said nothing. As the nursing notes said, he was mostly non-responsive. We were not to say anything to him about the accident, per family request. The family wanted to talk to him when they could get there, not before. But to Alan the absence said enough. He didn't know what it said, but it said enough.

Days went by.

Then Barbara came back. She still didn't say anything to him. He was supposed to be dying. He looked close… in a way. Maybe he couldn't take in the information, she said. It didn't seem like you could talk and have a conversation with him. Most of the time. The doctors had said weeks. Over 6 months had passed since then. We thought he had maybe days after admission. Weeks were going by since then.

I entered the room with morphine to ease his excessively rapid breathing. I was giving him a maximum dose for the orders in hand. I thought he was dying, and his presentations were extreme. I wanted his passing to be easy. His skin was hot and sweaty, his breath labored with his accessory muscles working hard to help him take in each inhalation. He was trying to sit up. His skin was pale and blotchy, his nails cyanotic. Olanzapine helped. He was stressed without it.

When I came back with the medicine, his body had changed from hot and sweaty, to cool. More signs. He was still breathing hard and was agitated. His quick change from feverishness to coolness, spoke (I thought) to a fast progression toward letting go of this life.

I gave the same anti-agitation medication that worked with him. I went to call Barbara and asked her how important it was for her to be here when her dad dies. She said she wanted to be there. I said, then, she better come over. I told Alan that she would be here soon, even if he didn't look like he could hear me. Hearing is the last sense that goes, it is believed.

When she showed up with her son and one other family member, not only did Alan look at ease, and with relatively good skin color, but his eyes were open and he was alert. What was it... 2 am? I had woken the family from their much needed sleep to come back and wait in exhaustion. They lived between visiting their dad in the hospice home, to alternately going to see their mom in the hospital. The family energy had brought Alan back.

Barbara had a deep chest cough. She had a great energy about her nonetheless. Her exhaustion was so great she almost couldn't recognize it any more. She, Ken (the aide), and I, chatted at length in the kitchen over tea. That is where we heard a lot of the story about the accident and how the wife was. *"Mom has given up,"* Barbara said. *"My son thinks it is selfish of her because she still has us."*

"People get tired;" I said, "Plus she knows she is losing her husband."

"This August will be their 70th ," Barbara said. "She is the kind of woman that didn't develop her independence. Me and my husband: We have our independent lives and we meet between. My parents are like one person. They are as if part of each other's limbs. What is better? Worse? I don't know, it's just the way we are."

I found out later that even before the accident, when Dawn was at home and Alan on hospice at VRH, that Dawn had pretty much lost her appetite and had stopped eating. She didn't know how to keep going without her husband.

"Yesterday the palliative care doctor came to talk to her and she asked to come here to inpatient hospice, but there were no beds," Barbara said.

Diane, the patient I had been grieving at the start of the shift, was dead. Her room was empty. Dove Room was open. I wondered if there was a waiting list on that room, and if Dawn could move in there. "Does she still want to come?" I asked. *"I don't know,"* Barbara said, *"That was yesterday."*

Ken and I spoke to the incomprehensibility of the pile-up of intense challenges that Barbara was going through. She shared with us other huge life events in her family, any of which alone might break someone. Barbara said, *"I could wring the necks of people who say, 'Well, it can't get much worse than that.' — It can."*

Before I left work that morning I sent a message to my boss and the administrator – Just in case they didn't know about the wife's desire yesterday for a bed at VRH. The daughter did not seem to be actively pursuing an opening; I think she was putting one foot in front of the other, and little more, at that point.

As I donned my 'tool belt' the next night, and put my reading glasses on my lower nose, Laurie — the RN going off evening shift — said, "There are two people in Giraffe Room. There is a new patient assigned to Dove Room, but we rolled the bed in with Alan. They are husband and wife."

Barbara was visiting in the Giraffe room, and chatted with me. The night before she had said she needed to let go blaming herself for her mother's condition.

"Did it all happen for this?" she said.

The two patients, now both mostly non-responsive, (apparently Dawn had a stroke in the last 24 hours and was not verbally engaging) had a calm about them that was a palpable difference to the sense of pressured waiting that Alan had held until now. Barbara said the transformation in her mom was also palpable from yesterday to today. Alan had been waiting for his wife.

The nursing report said that both had acknowledged each other's presence upon reunion. Barbara looked more at ease too. We all felt the change."The woman who died in Dove room made way for your Mom," I thought out loud. She made way for your Mom and Dad."

"I feel like I am in a soap opera," Barbara said.

"Life is short, Love is Long."
~ Dr. Patty Bilhartz Diblasio

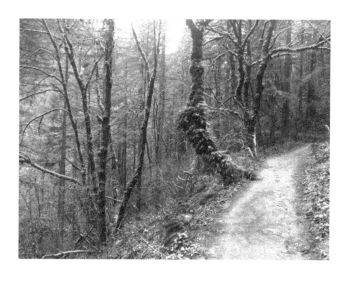

KINDNESS GROWS

From the first timid offering

Wrapped in tangled eloquence

To the silent touch

That stings and warms frozen hands

~ Rachel Houck, RN

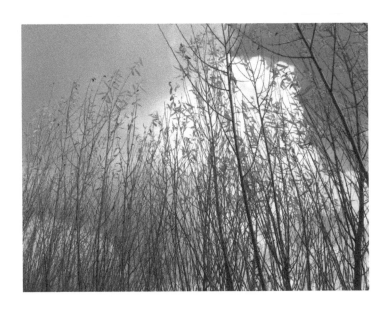

HER EYES

I am trying to think about how I can tell you about Erin
without describing her eyes.
I imagine my reader to be tired of being told about the depth of one's eyes.
Mouths, my brother says, express so much more in their curves and moods.

But for eyes today I am going to plead your patience,
because, as tired as I am after a full night's work,
and on my youngest daughter's 18th birthday,
as much as I want to get up refreshed to pull off her party after my sleep,
with a bonfire and 18 Chinese floating lanterns,
moving forward from my motherhood with children,
still, it is Erin's eyes that insist I write her story.

I wish I could draw them for you.
Or better have my now 18-year-old artist draw them.
A thickness of black outline without mascara or eye liner,
and the longest lashes I have seen, with a focus, bright and intent,
so wide that the eyes feel bigger than her emaciated body.
They focused almost constantly toward the ceiling slightly to her left.
They never closed and never blinked.
I started my shift being told her heart was no longer palpable in her wrists,
and that she was very close.

When she died three hours later with a room full of family characters —
one brother almost as cachectic as she, with a long black beard,
another with burns on both sides of his face,
others of varying ages and social engagement —
her focus did not release.

When the nursing aide did the post-mortem care,

her neck would not relax against the bed
even if the rest of her body was still warm and limp.
The intensity of direction remained.
Anza, the aide, was experienced about Life enough to not react impulsively.
But when a cool movement of air passed the back of her (Anza's) neck,
as she tried to put the body at rest, it shook the aide's serenity.
The eyes wouldn't close. Erin did not seem gone yet.
Anza lit a candle, said a prayer for Erin's release, and put on some soft music.

The tangible difference between the release of spirit from a dead body
comes in varying degrees.
When the spirit leaves the body it looks a mere shell,
if the spirit has not yet left, the person looks alive, just not breathing.
They look very still, or asleep, but not gone.
Just the heartbeat and breath is gone.

Erin's body was a skeleton coated in thin flesh.
Except for her eyes, she looked like the bones that hang in biology classes.
(Only her lower half was filled with fluid and puffed.)
Choose your most luscious cosmetic model, and they would want Erin's lashes.

I feel like I met a circus band last night, for which maybe Erin had been the
muse. Each family member, a new character in their own extraordinary way,
each present and connected around this woman
whom they described as the kindest one could know.
Each wearing scars of a hard life,
now softened in their love for their sister,
comforted in a home-like environment after a long hospital stay.

They were loud, raucous, told stories, laughed.
There was a kind of brute strength in everything they did.
I didn't know much of the patient's life story,
to say nothing of any of the other eight or nine in the room.
They told of their deceased father's history
which seemed to frame the others in the room, and fit the cavalry:

Apparently the father worked with the electric company.
The family said one day the dad was up on an electrical pole.
He called the main office
and told the controller to turn the power off for that pole.
The office said they did so. But they hadn't.
The father was electrocuted.

"He was thrown 35 feet," the son with the burnt face said.
"It went through his shoulder, down his leg and through his heel.
The medics said that if he hadn't cracked open his skull that he wouldn't have
survived — He got pressure-relief by cracking his head open."

The sister contributed that you didn't mess with this man's law.
"He would meet a complete stranger and say, 'What kind of dick-head are you?'"
The sister said that he could hold spark plugs
or unprotected electric cords after,
while the electricity was going through it, and it would do nothing to him.

I couldn't tell how much a fable had developed.
I had learned to listen to the incredulous with an openness to the unknown.

"When his good Priest friend asked him
if he might not want to make peace with his Lord, he said,
'Look, fella, I've done the dying thing;
I went to the devil and he didn't want me,
I went to heaven and they didn't want me there,
now I am back here stuck with your kind of God, and I don't want any of it.'
He lived another twenty years after his accident."

The family left soon after Erin died.
They left as unceremoniously as they arrived. The man with the scars winked.
"She would have been there for us if it had happened that way."

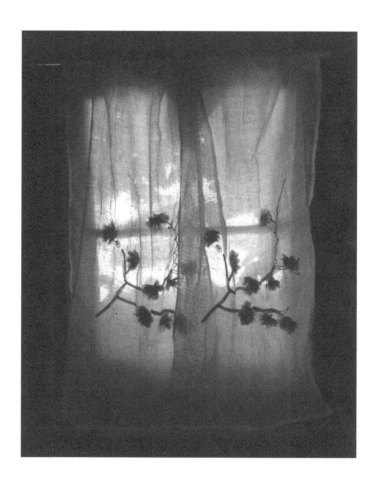

I WOULD HAVE

I would have
washed you with water from the creek and
lavender from the valley.

I would have
kissed you in turns.

I would have
brushed your hair with bone and
skin with linen.

I would have
placed pennies on your eyes.

I would have
laid you in furs and
feathers in your curls.

I would have
spoke, "God."

I would have
laced pearls 'round your neck and
one hand in the other.

I would have
stretched the sheet out flat.

I would have
rested my brow on yours and
my tears on your stillness.

I would have
held your hand.

I would have
smiled.

~ Scott Wilson, M.Div., BCC

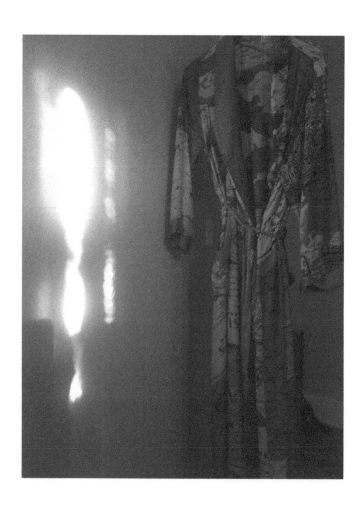

THE UPS MAN

She stood in her doorway, with her nightgown off one shoulder, her thick white hair past her neckline, half out of the combs that usually held the locks back, with a look of humble elegance.*"Would you get me a bite to eat?"* She asked the only person in the house who didn't seem to be in a hustle. It happened to be a man in a UPS uniform. It was 9:30 at night. He was kindly and responsive, and jumped on his task as if he had been waiting to be asked. When he arrived with a whole package of crackers and a banana, Juliana noted,*"I'm not that hungry!"*

"I was wondering if we could share."

The reason I knew the details above, even if I was not there, is that her figure in the doorway was not a new one to me. I put together the many versions of the story told by staff, and now the residents.

At that point she thought she was telling me a dream: *"He was the first person going by, and I knew I couldn't make it to the kitchen myself. So he brought me the crackers and banana, and sat down on the couch. I asked him if he worked here. 'No,' he said. I asked him if he had family here. 'No,' he said. 'Then what are you doing here? I asked him. 'I just parked in the lot and came in for a bite to eat.' 'This is not a weigh station,' I said to him. I was starting to get a funny feeling about it. I suppose I could have called the police. I didn't even think of it. He started to ask me about God. 'I'm not an authority on that! You should talk to a priest,' I told him."*

Still, apparently they did talk about God. My guess is that she had more thoughts to share on the subject than she gives herself credit for. Maybe precisely because she didn't consider herself an authority.

"We had a nice conversation," she said, *"But I still was feeling there was something wrong."*

This is one of the patients that wakes up at medication time, whatever the hour, and engages in conversation. She relishes interaction. She told me on another night that she had wanted to go to Juilliard — that she sang. She wanted to be a nurse… but instead she married and had kids. Not until now, she said, had she realized that she had not made choices for herself in her life.

"My babies were for me, though," she said, with a softness and longing, I thought. She spoke of being home as her highest aspiration now. She wanted to go home to live. *"I want to have coffee in the morning with my husband while reading the paper. I miss that. I know he can't take care of me,"* she said, crying. *"But what am I supposed to do now? Just wait to die?"*

She said she was embarrassed by how she acted when she had first arrived at VRH. She had fought it with every ounce of disempowered energy with which she felt overcome.

"I said I didn't want to be in this dump." I remember her snapping at me in the first weeks. It is hard to remember, with her softness and expressions of gratitude now. How can one underestimate the wrenching from home at one of the most vulnerable times, when not choosing it?

Tonight she continued telling her story about the man in the UPS uniform: *"That's when the nurse came in."* The nurse was ready to welcome the friend… No…the family member… No… did the resident know this man?… No… "You will be leaving," the nurse said to the man. *"Okay,"* he said casually while finishing his cracker. "No," the nurse interjected, "You will be leaving this minute, or I am calling the police." He left quickly.

The police came later. A report was filed. The man's license plate had been written down by the savvy nurse before he had driven off. If he showed up again, we were to call the police right away.

It turns out he had walked in with other family members on a busy night, and had gone unnoticed — except by Arthur, another alert resident who had been getting a snack at the same time the crackers were coming out. *"I knew he didn't belong here the moment my eye caught him,"* Arthur said.

As it turns out, the man came back the next day to apologize.

His mother-in-law had died at the home some time in the past — It was a place in which he felt comfortable on a lonely, hungry night. Juliana was calling it her nightmare. I debated whether I should tell her that it had really happened. If she was less cognitively aware, she might feel safer leaving it in the dream world. But she was very aware. Out of respect, I told her that it had not been a dream. She didn't believe me at first. I told her the measures being taken so it wouldn't happen again. I spent some time trying to empower her and get it out of the realm of intruders.

I was taken by the grace with which she handled the situation, and I told her so. *"He WAS good-looking,"* she said, with the secret smile a young girl keeps for the apples of her eye. Together we laughed.

When she took her second round of overnight medications, I apologized for not having brought a good-looking chap with me. She smiled dreamily and fell back to sleep.

© Ink by Anya Katrina Smith

LOVE IS LETTING GO OF FEAR

Some people are just annoying
Even as they're dying.
They push you away
Yet invite you back
To push you away again.
They make you feel small.
So they can feel big.
And you go along
Because they're failing.

Week after week
You reach out and serve
Yourself up on a platter
Knowing full well they will eat you alive.
It is, after all, how they matter.

Slowly but surely
They draw you back to the
Words of a younger you.
You're
Unlikeable
Wrong
Unworthy of love.
Words you now know to be
Mostly untrue.

Then one day
They surprise you by opening up.
They don't quite succeed
But they're trying.

So,
You return,
Bare,
Just as you are,
And rather than snub you
They see you
As worthy and
Good and
Easy to love.
It's what you've been all along.

~ Mary Brutsaert. LCSW

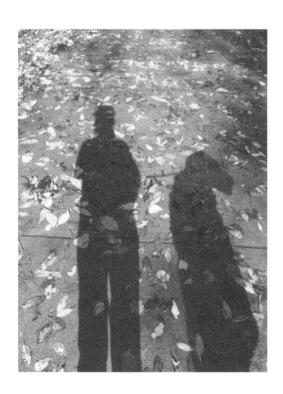

TEARS

One plastic cup of peanut m&ms. One plastic cup of peanut-butter m&m's — These are a new kind. So are the pretzel ones in the third cup. A black indelible pen was used to scribble a defining label on each cup.

Five large bags of m&m's sit on a low stool under the huge flat-screen TV he brought with him. His computer sits in the adjacent corner. Neatly placed around him are his personal items. "Where do you want me to leave this?" I asked him after emptying his urinal and wanting to leave it in reach.

"Right here is fine," he said, pointing to the center of the bedside table where his m&m's enticed. "I guess this will be your centerpiece," I said, knowing he had a sense of humor — Not knowing how good it was in nursing-practice.

"We'll put one single flower in it... or a straw," he said, as I turned to leave.

Even laughing took his breath away. He hardly dared move. His advanced arthritis contributed to his chosen spot in bed, as well as choosing a urinal over the pain of moving excruciatingly achy joints in getting up to the toilet or even to the bedside commode.

He cried as easily as he laughed in those days.

"My dream was to move to Florida and buy myself a mobile home. I did it. After sixty-five years in Vermont, I moved to Florida. I wasn't in a camp. I had my own piece of land." He said he lived there thirteen years. *"When I got sick, my family was still here. They wanted me to come back. It wasn't my choice."*

He had spent time painting on canvas in his Florida home. We arranged with the social worker for the paintings to get sent to him. They are on his wall now. Whatever critics say of a piece, Man and his art are one. I could see him in his paintings. I imagined him in his home.

"I handed my keys over to my neighbor. He bought the place." His face held its unchanged expression while tears streamed down on either side. The oxygen concentrator mumbled its motor. The TV dramatized the movie he had showing. I could hear the wind pressing the window. Still, it felt quiet enough to hear the tears fall.

He broke the silence:

"Take some m&m's before you go. People like the ones with peanut-butter. I'll have to get some more... Leave the door like the sign says. I asked my daughter to change the sign to leave it open six inches. I don't want to bother anyone with my TV."

The opposite side of the door did not have the updated sign with the six-inch instruction. "Six inches, huh?" I said. "Exactly? I'll change the sign on the other side too," I told him.

I taped a paper wound-measure-ruler onto the door and put an arrow pointing to the "6". I left the room laughing. He was laughing too.

"Hey!" he said, *"You left my door wide open!"*

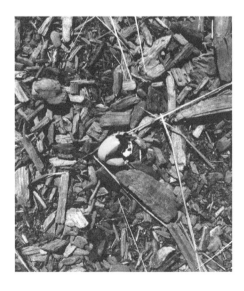

LOAVES AND FISHES

This is not
the age of information.

This is *not*
the age of information.

Forget the news,
and the radio,
and the blurred screen.

This is the time
of loaves
and fishes.

People are hungry
and one good word is bread
for a thousand.

~ David Whyte

Part Three

THE VALLEY OF KNOWLEDGE

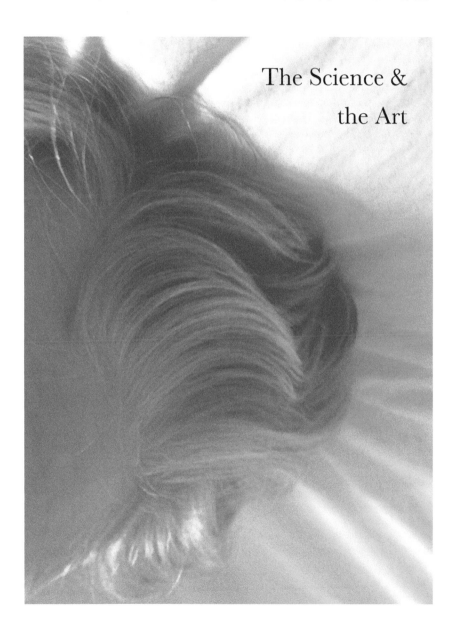

The Science &
the Art

THE DEFIBRILLATOR

Inside, I think Ken is a social worker. He just hasn't gotten there yet by license. He works as a nursing aide at Vermont Respite House. He lives in a humble cabin home off-grid in the Northeast Kingdom. He has a wood stove only, in the deep of Vermont winters. When he gets home he waits to warm up until the fire gets going. Thirty degrees Fahrenheit, or twenty degrees below zero, still the same. Then he has to be careful to not get his place overheated, while the couch holds the cold for hours.

He has a magic with people. He has a capacity to listen outside of himself and meet people where they are. That's what takes the loneliness away when you are with him. He has a way of taking life as it is, without distracting attention on himself, while also not forgetting to treat feelings with tenderness. He is committed to a life of preserving gentle connections with whomever is near. As such, he is present with death and dying.

A woman had arrived the day before. That was the night I learned the hard way how to deactivate an implanted defibrillator. The woman was fully alert. *"Is my cat bothering you?"* she asked. "No!" I said. One of the many lovely gifts of inpatient hospice homes is that there is room for your cat to stay, and for your dog to visit.

A few hours later:

"I am sorry to startle you awake; I brought your night medicine." She took her routine medications and went right back to sleep. I listened to the day's report. Regarding the new resident, the review said that she had declined turning off her implanted defibrillator. She wasn't ready for that. Moving-in had been enough for one day: No more big decisions until she settled in.

When people want hospice, they usually want to turn off their defibrillators. Pacemakers don't make a difference in prolonging death — Those turn themselves off. A pacemaker does not push a heart to beat after it stops, it just regulates the heart while it beats. A defibrillator gives electrical impulses to a stopped heart to get it going again. Generally in hospice we call in a specialist to turn the defibrillator off because people don't want to be jolted awake when they drift off quietly to die. When the woman declined turning it off today, we said we could address it tomorrow, when relieved from the heat of her moving transition.

When I write to you with other stories, I want you to see how death is natural, easy, after the work to get there. I want you to feel less scared by it after reading these stories, not freaked out. Also, the only way you are going to believe the more beautiful stories is if I tell you the whole picture of our experience, including the ones that are more difficult in which to see the redemption. Some stories are harder.

Ken was in hearing-distance and heard her yell, *"Help!"* It is like Ken to be not just waiting for call-bells in the staff room, but to have been where he was needed in hearing-distance at the moment. The nursing aides keep the pulse of the house. The nurses rely on them for this. We see that the heart of the house beats steady, but the aides catch the irregular heartbeats.

I think the patient said she needed a drink of water. When Ken tried to help her sit up to drink, she went limp. When I arrived, she looked like she was taking her last breaths. I went out for morphine and Lorazepam while the aides stayed with her, in case I was wrong and there was more time. When I came back, she was gone. We felt struck. "You'd think we would see more sudden deaths here," Ken said, "and that we would be more used to it — but it is actually rare." I had to agree with him. We were a bit shaken up.

Next we had to call the family. If we felt shook up, how would they feel? Then I remembered the defibrillator. I raced to the med room for the magnet put aside for this purpose, placed it over the defibrillator, realizing with loathing that I did not know the specifics of how to turn it off with the magnet. I told myself to use my common sense. I asked Francine, the second nursing aide who is getting her masters degree, and who has the gift of not losing natural intelligence, to please get on-line and try to find out how to use the magnet. She held her calm. I called the on-call administrator, who could not help me. I should have called the Medical Director but didn't think of it.

The patient's body was quiet. Fifteen minutes went by and there was still no activity. I took off the magnet, not realizing it had to stay on to keep the defibrillator off. I did the necessary assessments and pronounced her dead twenty minutes after her last breath. "I should call the family," I said. "We will clean her up so she is ready in case the family comes in," Ken said. I called the daughter. The daughter burst into open sobbing almost before I had finished telling her that her mother had passed suddenly. Already there was a feeling of unusual alarm in the home. Death is usually quiet, more like the river than thunder. But thunder walked in the door next. It was Ken telling me that the defibrillator was going off.

I pride myself in being calm in the face of high stress. I learned this as a child and have used it well professionally. But tonight I did not feel calm or collected. I knew I did not have a skill that was needed at hand — how to turn off that defibrillator. If I had not called the family, I would have felt a little better about timing. Having called the family, I envisioned them walking in to see their mother's body with the defibrillator going off, jerking the body whose turn it was to be quiet.

I needed to take care of it before they walked in the door, or if later, not fumble in their presence and add to their panic. I placed the magnet over the defibrillator, listened to its beep... (I have later learned that not all beep, but some do.) I still did not know to keep it on there, though in retrospect it seems obvious. I found out the next day in the quiet of my study, that I just needed to leave the magnet on. A pacemaker as well as a defibrillator's 'switch' gets turned off in the presence of strong magnetic energy, and turns back on when the magnet is taken off. Oh so obvious in hindsight without the mind-block of stress. *"It's easy when you know how,"* Sara used to say to me. (The woman who *'wouldn't do anything except for sitt'n still'*, but got up and caught the child from falling). After an hour, the electric shocks stopped on their own, before the family arrived, and finally the body quieted down.

Death has many unpredictable components. But the body not being quiet after death was not in our repertoire of the unpredictable. I think one copes by relying on the reliable to handle the unreliable. There is much unknown to cope with in our work. What we had relied on, got upset.

On the next night, when a different family pushed the wheelchair-access button on our locked doors and entered the house (because we had forgotten to push a power button to confirm the locking), we still held the ghost of edginess in wondering if living people could now walk through locked doors quietly, just like dead bodies could now re-activate.

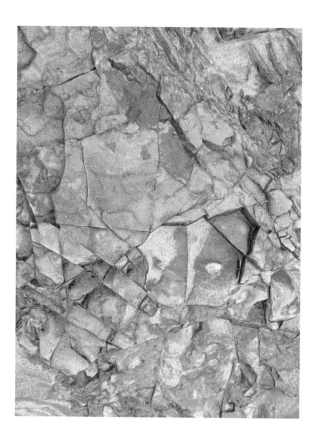

THE 'Y' DANCE

Mickey Tango and I arrived at VRH at 6:30 pm.
The dining room table was moved aside.
Juliana was sitting in her wheelchair with her husband sitting next to her.

"We liked the jitterbug," he said.

Since Juliana was not able, the husband acquiesced to dancing a jitterbug
with me,
to music on a You Tube video connected to Arthur's speakers.

Arthur was the person who had recognized the UPS man as a stranger a month
ago. He had lived ten years in *San Miguel de Allende* in Mexico
(where I lived for a bit as a girl).
He was dying of colon cancer at VRH.

Juliana was the woman who had received the UPS man.

"Do you know the Y dance?" the husband asked me after dancing the jitterbug,
and saying he couldn't breathe anymore. "No," I said truthfully.

"Do you want me to show you?" he asked.

We got onto the dance floor and into a close embrace,
as Michael and I had done for our mini Argentine Tango performance that
night
for Juliana and her husband and Arthur and company.

"A little closer," the husband said.

I was used to getting close to tango dancers, so I didn't find it too strange
that he asked that...
Or if I did, a little closer when life is short is not all so bad in good company.

"Why dance?" he said, and sat down. That was the Y dance.

Dreamily as Juliana dozed off to sleep that night,
She talked softly with a smile on her face, about dance and love.

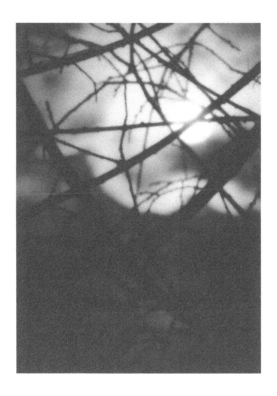

BREATH

When Elizabeth's husband was up for the second time with bad ankle cramps, after already having taken Ibuprofen for his right arm post-surgical pain (family being almost as much a part of the treatment plan as our patients) it felt natural to offer an oil leg massage. Especially when I had just put the massage oil down for the man across the hall who was an athlete and was taking days to die after everyone thought he was taking his last breaths and that it would be hours.

He and Elizabeth had gotten married one month after I was born, fifty-two years ago. Monday would be their anniversary. I saw the photo in the light he turned on for a brief moment. In the dark I never did see his present aged face. In the photo he and his bride had reddish hair. They were very young. She had spice and independence in her attitude and thin frame. He had mojo. The groom was well built from work. His eyes had direction. Both the wife and husband had simultaneously an independence of spirit and a togetherness that attracted me. I commented on her energy.

"She was always like that," he said.

She didn't really look that different in bed tonight. She was both soft and feisty.

It turns out that he went into the Navy at age eighteen. He left it at some point in adulthood after years of service, opened a gasoline station in Vermont, and then went back into the Navy. He said he missed it when he was away from it. He spent his life there fixing jets. *"I had the kind of job that I could enjoy every day. I fixed airplanes, cars — anything. I would get a motor and after a day's work it was purring. That was the reward of the day."* I could hear the intelligence and mastery in his voice. He said he had retired from engines. *"I am too old now."*

His ankle was twitching. *"I left my quinine home. I didn't think it would bother me tonight, but I mowed for the first time this spring and that is probably why."* His spirit did not seem old. In the dark, as his wife slept, I could hear his 18-year-old self. He said they met in a restaurant, he and Elizabeth. Unexpectedly. He knew at first sight that he wanted her as his wife. I asked him if she was hard to win over.

"Of course," he said, *"She is Irish. I am French. I used to have an awful accent. I learned English when I was thirteen. She called me 'Frenchie 'from that point on."*

I asked him how he had won her love. *"I kept working at it,"* he said simply.

He had a grace of receiving and giving back. The men in my life are good at being simple and straightforward. My experiences feel complex, and my moods to match. This man shared his life story openly as his twitching ebbed away. His wife was not hard-of-hearing in the bed next to his pull-out couch, though she was minimally responsive. She got the gift of reminiscing as she heard her husband talk about her.

Hearing, it is said, is the last sense that goes before dying. It is easy to forget that a dying person is still listening, at one level or another. In nursing school times, when I lay on the floor on my back after fainting from witnessing a knee surgery with the patient awake on local anesthesia, I had the experience of hearing everyone around me while not looking conscious. That is how I imagine people when they lie dying and looking unconscious. If they are unconscious, remember hearing things in your dreams and your dreams changing to fit what you hear. You are heard. Your loved one may want quiet for their process, or they may hunger for your words when closure is not complete. If you are so inspired, laugh and tell each other stories of your life. It will give to two primal dying needs: One, *"I must have done okay if they have good memories,"* Another: *"My family must be okay if they are laughing and happy. I may rest at ease."*

The cat too was relaxed as I closed the screen door for rooms with pets. The family went to sleep breathing in the shadows. When she dies, her breathing won't so much stop, as breathe into existence.

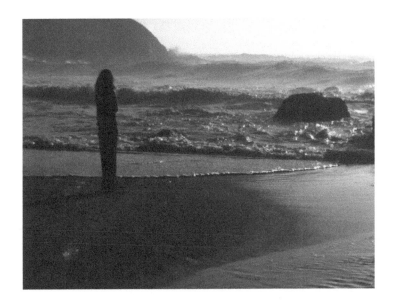

FIND

I will find you again my love,
in This Death or The Next.

After all, we have
found each other
once before—after
how many re-births of forgetting?

Do not
fret, much
about this
distancing goodbye,

spirits that have loved will
always be intertwined.

Let go of my hand, love
and listen for my voice upon the horizon.

Take a step and feel
this well-worn path to our returning.

~ Scott Wilson, M.Div., BCC

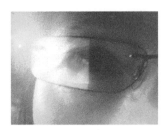

Our deepest fear is not that we are inadequate.
Our deepest fear is that we are powerful beyond measure.
It is our light not our darkness that frightens us most.
We ask ourselves who am I to be brilliant, gorgeous, talented, and fabulous?
Actually, who are you not to be?
You playing small does not serve the world.
There is nothing enlightened about shrinking
so that other people don't feel insecure around you.
We were born to make manifest the glory that is within us.
It is not just in some of us, it is in everyone.
And as we let our own light shine,
we unconsciously give other people permission to do the same.
As we are liberated from our own fear,
our presence automatically liberates others.

~ Marianne Williamson in *A Return to Love*

LOVING

"I didn't ever realize until now that nothing I did in my life was for myself... I wanted to go to Juilliard to sing. I wanted to be a nurse... Instead I got married. My babies were for me, though."

That's Juliana — the woman who welcomed the UPS man, and the woman who asked Michael and I to dance for her. She said she had danced from high school *"until I couldn't breathe any more."* She hated to see people smoking. She had a lot of remorse about that. Even if she had quit fifteen years ago when she got very sick. Maybe that is when she was first diagnosed with emphysema.

I went away for the weekend to visit my brother and daughter, and when I came back, Juliana was dead. So was Arthur; so was Elizabeth. Arthur was the guy who lent us his speakers when we danced at VRH. Elizabeth was the wife of the man who repaired motors and had ankle spasms... I miss them all. There was a story that I was going to write about Elizabeth and her mom, her mom who died a long time ago. But it is gone. The stories keep coming.

This morning it is Juliana again who is boring her consciousness into mine: In the period of time around when the UPS man visited, she was her happy self. She still had a lot to give. When she had first arrived, she was unhappy with herself, if you remember, and unhappy with everyone around her — which is what happens when we are unhappy with ourselves, of course.

Closer toward the end of her life she came back to the miserableness. Her life role was Giver: to Husband, to Children, to Family, to Neighbors. Why then in her last days did she become so bitter, so miserable, so tormented at the end of her stay at VRH?

She became demanding that her husband be called very late at night. When the evening nurse asked her if she was sure she wanted us to wake him at such a late hour, she said, *"Yes I do! If I have to go through this, then he does too."*

The day staff said she yelled persistently over the weekend. When Ken (the aide) told her gently that her husband would be in soon, and that her yelling was disturbing other patients, she hollered that she didn't care, without pause for reflection or delay in consideration.

She couldn't delay any more. She couldn't consider any more someone else's needs above her own. It was her turn, she said. The family was exhausted. After months of doting on her, desperately trying to give back all they received, in the end they were home when she died. Completely worn out. Nothing could fill Juliana up. No amount of attention and love. It almost seemed that she wanted in the end what she had not dared ask all her life. By then there was such a back-log, that bitterness and resentment and hunger and desire and longing and despair consumed her. She hated herself for it, but she couldn't help herself, it seemed.

Her body mirrored her psyche... as it does. At first she felt like she would never die, no matter how hard she wished it. The morphine was taking care of her shortness of breath remarkably, without even breakthrough episodes for the most part — for a while. She almost looked at times like she didn't belong at an inpatient hospice unit. We kept checking in on her status to see if she was one of the people to be discharged... Until we would see how weak and sick she was behind the mask of comfort that the drugs so remarkably upheld.

Then she got thrush; white fungal patches in her mouth and down her throat. She was in miserable condition. Nystatin solution, an anti-fungal swish-and-swallow rinse, took the patches away. It didn't stop there. Her mouth and throat became red and raw. Then it ulcered. Coating it with oil helped the excessive dryness. Cooking oil (avocado oil is my favorite) lasts longer on dry mouth than water or Biotene on mouth swabs. Lidocaine oral solution helped to numb her discomfort. Anxiousness, sense of helplessness, and misery went from frequent to persistent.

The night before going to Boston I was determined she was not going to have a night of unrelieved pain. It took 50mg of morphine over the night, along with 5mg Zyprexa for heightened angst, before she rested at ease. Her mouth and lungs were filled with infection. She didn't want antibiotics because she did not want to prolong her life. She coughed up green, thick, vile sputum. The ulcers grew with the increased secretions.

One of the wise and mature nurses said that she was spitting up all the vileness of her life. It seemed to me that she had swallowed what came down in her life. Her practice was to push it down, not nourish herself, we thought.

Giving gives back, but holding in gives out. Nurses understand this, when we understand ourselves, to monitor the trap of giving out of balance. Now she was spitting it out: All the poison she had harbored. She gave. She loved others. She took care of people, while holding back receiving fully from her deepest self and capacity. Her voice and song got drowned. Her possible career never happened.

How do we fool ourselves that it is giving to be silent? What keeps us from realizing and listening to ourselves? What are we afraid of in holding back? *"Be what you is because if you ain't what you is, then you is what you ain't."* Juliana paved the way for me and for others to remember to sing. To care for others, and to also allow ourselves to be cared for. And to follow our dreams.

We believed that she did spit it all up in the end. That her spirit is free now. To hear and to play her music. To love and to be loved.

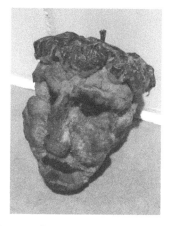

© Courtesy of SaraDowningPhotography.com

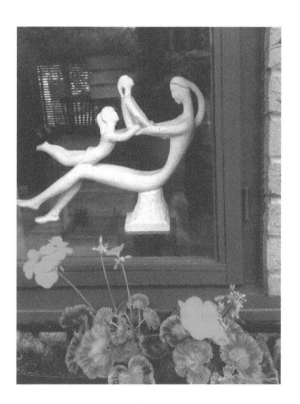

WELCOME HOME

If you are in your teens and trying to let go your mom connection, FYI you may still be calling her when you are 98-years-old.

Maybe more importantly, it may be your mom who welcomes you into what comes after death.

If you are a mom like me, wondering what your role is going to be with your now 18-year-old who has the sweetest boyfriend known, and her dad's house is closer to him than mine, tell me that mom-hood does not end here.

She helped remind me that herself today when she called. She was elated to tell me that Dylan (her boyfriend) hung posters from the roof of his house. The posters read, *"Will you go to the Prom with me?"* One of Anya's places closest to heaven — in addition to Dylan's arms — is on the rooftop of our family home.

Anya said the *"yes"* sign was on one side of the roof. The *"no"* sign was in black, with a sad face, and was on the floor by the garage. It didn't matter that the *"yes"* was harder to reach because it was high. The rose petals that were strewn up to the doorway, the bouquet of red roses in her sweetheart's hands when he opened the door, made it difficult to answer right away in any way, with Anya's emotions smiling so wide and her heart so full.

Some people call their mothers all their lives. (Well, except maybe in the years they need to establish their individual identity.) Some aging people call their mothers throughout their debilitating years.

Others are like Coreena, at ninety-eight years old, who called her mom days before she died. It was not usual for Coreena to call for her mother, said her daughter-in-law Pauline. Coreena's eyes were usually closed now. Her previously difficult words to comprehend were now clearly audible. *"Mother, Mother, Mother."*

Dying people often look up into a corner of their bedroom ceiling. They speak names in an apparent trance-like state, mumble, often inaudibly. It is a private time in which they appear to be connected to their ancestors. There is no room for a nurse there, beyond giving them space and comfort to pursue their communications in an unknown world to us. It is a world beyond what we can understand.

With Pauline and Coreena there was more sharing and less mystery. Pauline said that Coreena was her mom in all ways — not just an in-law. They could talk about anything, she said. They were best friends every day.

Coreena, still in her audible voice, told Pauline what her mother was telling her: *"She says it is beautiful. She says it is beautiful. She says it is beautiful. She says I should go."* Her words were simple and repeated. *"I think it is true. They should kill me."*

It is said that if we knew what it was like post-death, that we would not be able to bear waiting for it, and we would kill ourselves instantly. — That is how I understood Coreena's wish.

Pauline said that Coreena had a son who was a favorite of hers, and that the son would not come to see her. Pauline felt that Coreena was waiting for her son to come, before she let herself die. The son was not coming, it seemed, no matter how many times or ways Pauline begged him — or gave him space, or any support received from her wonderful social worker on the team. Coreena's mom was telling her that she should come to pass anyway; that it was okay.

Pauline was a strikingly beautiful young woman. Self-composed in a way unexpected in a grieving world. Her face did not strain as she cried. I only knew she was crying in the dark because she was wiping her tears. I felt a bit like an intruder. I didn't feel that Pauline needed me. Nor Coreena. I sat as witness, no more. The sounds of the house felt distant. That of our hearts felt loud.

ABODE

Where does the hand that touched our travail
go to rest?
Where do the eyes that witnessed our tears
find something else to see?

Oh that you may travel in peace you brave one!
You who always walked alone but always beside us.
May you find the secret place of songbirds
who rest their song.
May you take refuge in clefts of mountains
that never tremble.
May you know solace as your sister
like rain in a dry land.

~ Kim Bakondi, MSW, CSWA
(Written for Janine Carranza, author.)

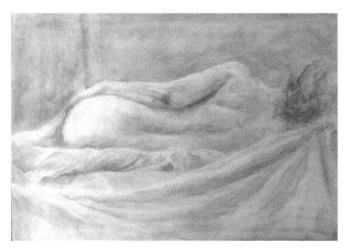

© Drawing by Anya Katrina Smith

A WRINKLE IN TIME
WITH GEORGE CLOONEY

Dreams. Angelina wakes every night panicked. She's the woman who makes me think of one of the witches in A Wrinkle in Time: A quick word, an easy a wink. "I love you," I tell her.

"Don't get caught," she says, or, *"I like it when you talk dirty."*

Another night she quipped: *"The town was so small, the hooker was a virgin."* *"It is good to laugh, isn't it? Just don't wet your pants."* No one spoke better to describing the chocolate nutrition drinks we offer: *"Chocolate is good when chocolate is good, but the rest of the time it isn't. It doesn't make much sense, but neither do I."*

She's the gal with a huge portrait of George Clooney facing opposite her bed. Kate and Laurie (the evening nurses) figured out how to get Make a Wish Foundation have George Clooney call her. It took months, but it happened. Her memory and communication is too fractioned for me to get a picture of how the call went. She didn't let anyone forget that she and George Clooney have their birthdays in the same month. This month, actually—May. We think Angelina will make one more birthday. Who knows. Who ever knows.

Her dreams haunt her. Her laughter and jokes can no longer hide the Nazis and the police and the child dreams that torment her. This morning the case manager said she'll talk to the daughter and call for a psych consult.

"Why does it happen?" Angelina asked.

"Well, sometimes when people have somewhere in their history experiences of having something or someone taking you over, feeling small and disempowered and scared in a profound way for too long a time, it comes back to you in nightmares after it is past."

"*Yeah,*" she said.

"Would that fit you?"

"*Yeah,*" she said.

That might have been the longest and most serious conversation I ever got with Angelina. She was the gal with the quips, not the sit-me-down and chat-and-share stuff.

I have nightmares too, of my own type. Last night, a tsunami was hitting a building with a slanted glass wall of windows. The building was holding up and not giving-in to the pressure of the waves. People from the beach were getting thrown up and flattened against the glass. It became a trance-like live movie screen to those inside the building, of people's deaths. Once the wave passed, those who had been able to hold their breaths not knocked unconscious, could be peeled off the glass and saved. My job was to take deep breaths inside the building and go out into the water to peel people away from the glass as soon as they hit, to try to save some of them.

The waves kept coming; I made trip after trip, pulling people away from the glass. It is all so clear, I feel like I am having the dream as I write it hours later. At one point my mother came as a tourist, cheerfully in pretty clothes, holding a little girl's hand and oblivious to the calamity. Then as some water hit her face and woke her to what was happening, I called to her and told her to go back up the trail she had just walked down.

The rest of the dream was of me taking trip after trip, wondering if the waves or my physical strength would give up first. At what point should I stop? In the attempt to help one more person, and chance that I would be the one dying against the glass, I had to ask myself if it was so smart or even honorable to drown trying to help a drowning person.

One month later: Angelina, as far as I know, is still at VRH. I am not. I am transitioning to the sunshine — day shift. In the circadian rhythm with more people. It is a new world into family's homes. Has Angelina welcomed yet her new world? I have not called to find out. Or read the obituaries.

Like the witches in A Wrinkle in Time, she is unforgettable. I can see her ever so soft white skin with just a touch of pink. Her sharp eyes and wry smile. Her sad face despite its laughter. Calling someone "cute" can be patronizing or less than respectful to their maturity. It can also be real. She was a damn cute master of some magical world.

I hope George Clooney charmed her. Even if she can't remember it. If he could have visited her instead of called her, she would have charmed him. Maybe she still instilled her charm on the phone, if he was present enough to have really talked to her. She got a box of cookies in his name a while later.

One more wrinkle in time.

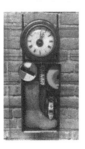

© Ana Durley

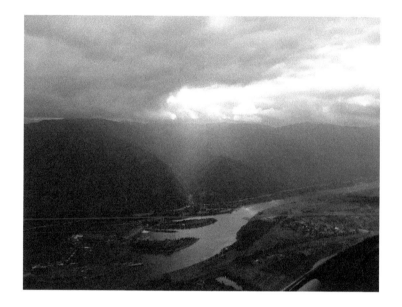

DYING IS HARD WORK

I wonder if everyone is afraid of dying
and we are all working to come to peace.

I wonder, when think we are not afraid,
if we will be when we face it more closely for ourselves.
I fear not having a chance to make it better anymore,
but also this moment is good enough as it is for now.
Loving now is the aim,
or minimally taking the courage to be with now,
however hard or dark or painful it reflects.

One day it will be my daughters' and your offspring's turn
to carry the torch for tomorrow without our physical help today.
Still, even then, one doesn't run out of chances to improve and to be.
Growth can happen on any plane, before and after death,
though this plane is a particularly potent and precious petri dish for growth.
It is all one: heaven and hell happens here
as much as love and joy and pain happens in the hereafter,
while the material challenge of life dares us
to make sure all is a metaphor for the spiritual and not a dependency or abuse.

I am still afraid in moments, and guess I will be again.
But courage isn't courage without fear.
If we don't feel fear, then we don't call on our courage.
My personal coping to the ugly is by trying to make things better
while finding gratitude in what is present.

Sometimes life's path feels inspired.
Sometimes it feels like putting one foot in front of the other,
or just stopping in the rain.

Until the light shines brightly again and new paths expose themselves
in grace from unexpected places and open people,
while vulnerably trusting enough to not drink darkness,
and then courageously stepping into exposure.

I wonder if, underneath, everyone is somewhere afraid of dying,
except for the moment when we are ready for the release of it,
and the moment we are present in the oneness.

Or maybe we are all afraid of living
until the moment we are ready to be released into its oneness.

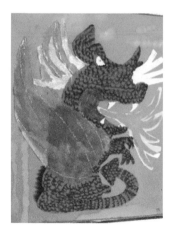

© Art by Samantha Carranza

TRYING TO DIE

Arthur was Arthur. I am not even sure if I have a story to tell you about him. Except that, as I sit in the sunshine between my old job at VRH and my new one coming up taking care of patients in their homes… It is him of whom I am thinking. He is already gone, as I mentioned before in another portrait, after sharing his speakers with us for the tango and "Y" dance at a moment when he felt more social than usual.

Maybe I am thinking of him because he spent many of his late adult years in Mexico — in a city I lived in as a girl for a little while, San Miguel de Allende. Sitting now on a café deck with hibiscus tea and feeling the sunshine on my arm and leg, with air moving just enough to feel its freshness, as if at a Mexican café, it is he who comes to mind.

He blended with the environment. He was quiet. He wanted to die as soon as possible once he could not sit in cafés anymore. Between wanting to die faster, and food making him sick, he decided to stop eating. He continued to drink fluids. If he thought he could die on command and in short order, the fluids he chose to continue drinking delayed that. We can live for months on just fluids. Even if he had chosen no fluids as well, he could have lived for weeks.

I have said that we have control over our deaths. I have said that feeling we do not have control over death,when all of us have to die sooner or later, is one of our greatest fears. I have said that we make our own signature right to the end. Arthur would have told me that I was lying. It was many a time that he said he was going to die before the end of the day. And didn't, to his very great dismay. He said he was desperate to die. But days and weeks and even months went by before he and his body let go. As Ken (the aide) said, every one of the sixty-plus days that Arthur counted and tried to predict, were days of singular focus and intention. He didn't smoke, he didn't eat, he didn't engage almost at all with staff, after the 'Y' dance. He did relish his fluids. When we went into his room, we were excused before five minutes were up. Very courteously. But excused all the same. He seemed to not want to distract the process. It was almost as if in his staring match with death, maybe he could will it.

He worked at conducting his care to the last inch. An orchestration to the minutest detail when possible. He seemed to seek cerebral manipulation as a friend. He wedded that struggle and reward for what it was.

In the end who knows. Maybe his will did win. Or did he finally let go?

Maybe both.

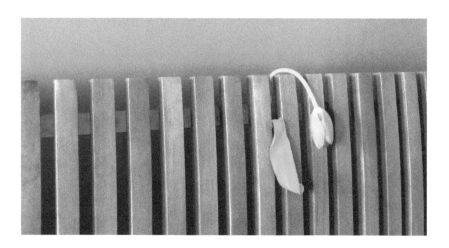

ANNA

Time is moving on. I have not told you about Anna. Sometimes the memories are so much a part of me that it feels as if I have already written them. Many I have not.

I have moved my hospice work into people's homes, outside of inpatient care. Now the patient is more boss than ever. That is why I moved into homes. (And to get off night shift after six years.) My hope is that the patient at home has an optimal chance of running their health and life, and that reign of the medical profession over vulnerable people may be kept in check. At your home you are at the helm. Healing needs helpers but comes ultimately from the sick person's path, not a professional's.

Anna, however, was boss at Vermont Respite House when she was there. She held a small dominion in her room. It was a world unto itself. She and her belongings and her books and her keen mind and her hooked rugs. She had been in a rug-hooking group and had become an refined artist in subtlety of color gradations. She had to send her rugging and literature books home with her daughter because she didn't have room for them. And her endurance for getting through the pages of a book was diminishing.

"You tell people you are dying and trying to get rid of stuff, and this is what they bring you. (She showed me her latest gift.) Now I need to find someone who wants it more than I do, which is hard because I like it."

She was a teacher in profession and at heart. Harry Potter had been an inspiration to her for her students.

"Harry Potter has invited people into the world of reading who before now have never read a chapter-book. It has introduced thousands of people to the magic world of storytelling and imagination."

She loved books and hooked rugs and gardens. She watched the life of the grounds outside her window. She had left her garden at home. She was the person who objected to some red plants in green pots out her window, instructing the hospice gardeners to please move them. They are now replaced with green foliage.

In the early morning before leaving the night shift, I would copy Anna a poem, or a saying, or a small intrigue of some sort, tape it to the end-point door, for her daily walk down the hall. She went inch by inch, one step at a time, as she held the railing that lined the walls for this purpose. I wanted to give her a hug in reward for her diligence and positive embrace on life.

Educated without superiority. Intelligent without arrogance. Dignified without separateness. Loving without control. Wise without self-righteousness. Beautiful without self-consciousness. Soft without debility. Strong without muscle.

That is Anna.

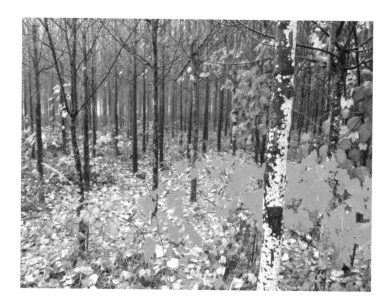

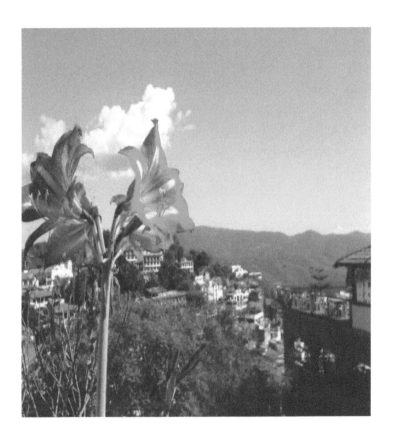

THE GAP

Thatched red brick rooftops. The stillness of the mausoleums, layered over each other. Encircled cluttered buildings poured over mounds and winding cobbled streets. A silver city amidst old mines, drenched with aged dreams of wealth.

My grandfather standing as one king of these imaginings. While my grandmother built a business and brought home the regular income. His fine original furniture for prestigious people brought in chunks of money that sometimes helped if he wasn't gambling it into the mines. His love of women was small to that for his wife whom he called the most beautiful woman on which his eyes had set. Katrina, 'the elegant one,' is the name now carried forward to our youngest daughter.

His charm and humor matched the Charlie Chaplin poster framed in the open room. It was a picture of himself dressed up and acting like Charlie. *"Cómicos también tienen tristeza,"* he would remind. He reminded us often that behind laughter is also tears.

The casket was of dark satin gray heavy metal. Silver-colored glossy curling decorations, with the impression of stainless steel, now suddenly sounding like plastic when hammered away. A crowd of people in black standing after a heavy rainfall.

First the mass with the church-full of people who loved and had relied on the man who took care of them. Then the procession, a long walk on the cobbled stone streets. Now the standing in the moist air waiting to see if the casket could be forced into the opening built in times when the caskets were made of wood. It was too large for the old openings. No one had measured, feeling safe in the long-ago secured place for this time. (You wouldn't know the dead man's competent sister ran a funeral home.) My youngest brother stood aghast.

The body under the glass of the now torn-away cover to the casket, was our father's. He can look out now. Of course he could anyway. In *Santa Lucía de La Sierra*, looking out was his life. As on the night he took me for our moon-walk in the high altitude where the moon's pregnant light and its earth were together. Where he and I were father and daughter with the deep breaths of pure air that cooled the spirit.

What do tears do? Except be. And maybe tell him from afar how dear he is to us. And then not be so far. He must be closer than ever now.

Though he can no longer help me across the ravine as I carry the calf hung across my shoulders, taking it back to its mother. Or rest his strong sculptured hands on my knee on the long trips across the country between the work in the mountains and my grandmother's house, his mother's home. Or grab the broken mercury thermometer from me as a little girl when I bit it in delirium, and rinse my mouth out with the urgency that only a father has for his daughter.

A young woman translates from English to Spanish the letter written in memory of the younger years teaching in an American school in Veracruz, Mexico. She stops where Jim, the teacher remembering *El Profesor* (as he was called), speaks of the young people Dad tutored and helped pivot and re-direct at critical junctures. *"I was one of those kids,"* she interrupts through tears. The letter found its place when one wondered if the hacking of the casket was a purification of a simple life remembered for its integrity, or a disruption to the sanctity of the occasion.

Finding a printer in town to print the words of this letter on that Sunday in a city not designed for the efficiency of business people, had trekked me through the old paths my dad and I had walked in some of my most impressionable years, through the parts of the market that fed the poor, not just those who could afford the upscale markets, down the tunneled walks where my grandmother knew to find the choicest fruits and vegetables for her table with the bright yellow tablecloth and hand-patted tortillas that puffed up without a single air-hole to keep them from pillowing on the *comal*. (An art I never mastered, though tried.)

Now reading the translation into Spanish of the copy that had been printed in an isolated tiny room where there was internet access, a public printer, and a long line to wait, we stood with the corpse of the man who lived, in many ways, as the villagers. No running water, no plumbing, no electricity. He lived in a home like theirs. In a town where doctors tired. No place to buy an ice cream cone or much else. Beer and Coke, yes. Candy and soap and *frijoles* and oil and salt and sugar, yes. No internet access. No social venues for intellectual pursuits. Unless you joined *El Profesor's* story-reading groups or bible study classes. Traditional regular social gatherings of music and prayer, and celebration, yes.

I thought Papi (that's what his children called him) always wanted to be a Doctor. Maybe he did before. But when he taught himself the care needed in the village from my nursing books, and our brother's medical school books, including IV's and birthing, hospice and treatments for plagues, he corrected me, saying with defensive emphasis, *"I am a teacher."*

Such is the Masters in Education he got at Columbia University. *"El Profesor"* remained his name into the days and years he spent in medicine, replacing the classroom days in local schools, but never completely replacing the hours pulled aside for a lesson someone needed in their academia.

Dad knew how to bring out inner knowledge, strength and wisdom. Learning new things brings out our insecurities and ignorance, but having *El Prófe Rey* as a teacher was about feeling safe to venture beyond the comfort zone.

He knew suffering, and as such understood it, and wanted to give relief to others. His compassion was accessible. When someone was in need, his gentleness knew how to touch where it most hurt. His face was soft. His nose flattened against his face like his ancestors. His hands well-built and skilled. His skin dark with its copper hue from the sun. His silver hair thick and handsome like his mother's.

He told us with a wink, of the young North American waitress who commended him on his highlights, assuming they came from a beauty salon. Dad had a good barber, but that is all his hair had seen. He could have been an American model with the Latin allure. But it was the stars and the wind and the poor people who saw his beauty in daily living.

Most women who met him, from age three to one-hundred, were in love with him. He didn't believe any one of them would have him.

The woman whom he had loved years ago, who birthed his six children, was long gone. The other women remained equal mysteries to him.

Papi is with his mother now, who understood him. He said he was not like the Mexicans, and not like the North Americans. He was most at home in his mother's kitchen, at a patient's bedside, reading a book, listening to classical music, helping a student progress his or her life, or taking a long walk in his village. The village that was so close to the stars you could reach up and almost touch them. He did so, I believe, on the night of his last walk.

Dad didn't want to have to be taken care of when he was old. He knew what that entailed. He gave that gift to his mother, and to countless others. He was last seen conscious on his evening walk on the same streets that he introduced to me over thirty years ago in the high altitude of the *Sierra Madre* in *Jalisco*. The next morning he was unconscious from a pervasive stroke. Four days later he was released of the burdens of this world.

Flying out to Mexico City for the funeral, I was scared. I could not dispel the event of my friend's brother being hung from a tree central to the townsfolk, by drug cartel clans, where Papi used to teach, after the family handed over $10,000 that the family did not have. During the funeral procession another friend told me of the men taken randomly from their store in this hometown *Taxco*, only weeks before, never to return.

My family was right in saying I had to go to the funeral, but nothing was feeling safe or smooth or easy or natural or practical about it. Except when my brother somehow unexpectedly got first class seats on his flights — As a tease from Dad, we thought.

My oldest brother looks after everyone else before himself (just like his dad).Dad loved to tell the story of how he himself got bumped accidentally to first class. He had the same teasing wink as if he had spent time highlighting his hair, when in actuality his world saw little of material luxury. My brother Todd felt as if Dad was winking at him again when it was Todd's turn on his way to Dad's funeral.

It was hard to invite Dad into our lives away from Mexico. He was never really at home in this country, as much as he was beloved here. He chose the mountains where he could re-connect to his integrity, I thought, in a pained world. With his absence in his children's lives, he said at a commemoration ceremony at Earlham College where he got his BA:

"May it be a consolation to them [my children] that they have been my inspiration."

As we flew to Mexico City, we were aware of others from divers parts of the country, flying toward the same destination, while flights and seats coincided as if from a pre-meditated plan greater than our own tedious controls.

The casket finally fit in the cement opening after much shoving from the men. It might have been the beautiful wood casket that was in the basement of our family home — made, we think, by his father who was an accomplished woodsmith.

We thought it fit Dad, but that Dad's brothers and sister never did quite understand how Dad had not pursued the material rewards of life after his good education and opportunities. They saw it as an honor to give him a fancy casket. It did not match his life, we thought, but it did match their love in wanting only their best for him.

Despite all, the casket with Dad in it, found its own way to simplicity. A random board for a door was jammed over the opening once the casket was finally in. It was a plain and old board; no marking on it. Memory told the family whose body was behind which opening of the mausoleum, one above the other behind the concrete: His Mother, His Father... *Doña Cata*... His Brother. Our spots are designated there too, without our names. We might fit in that slot or we might not. Our turn is next.

For now our turn is here.

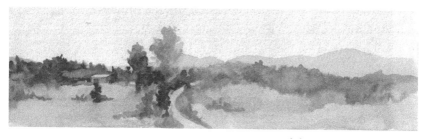

© Ink by Anya Katrina Smith

THE GAP

I'm at our place by the river in the woods.
In the absence of his physical presence is a gap.
A gap too large to measure or contain or define.
It brings to mind the falling
not of grace
but of an immeasurable tree.
And a habitat
for the many new plants and shoots
now growing in the fertile soil
that has developed over all these years
from its leaves and limbs falling and decomposing.
Now it's for you and me:
To fill
from what is left with us...
Until we leave a gap.
The tears, the wrenching open.
Where the children flourish.

~ Anonymous

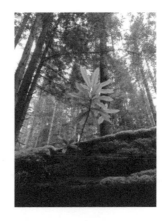

Dear Rey... Go in peace, my friend.

It is with a very heavy heart that I find myself writing this note and unable to be with your family and friends as they gather in your beloved Taxco to give final tribute to all that you have accomplished in your life, as a father, a mentor, and a friend.

You were my mentor... having a lasting and positive impact on a very young, new teacher that you recruited to join you in Veracruz so many years ago, introducing me to your chosen lifestyle of living in a small rural village, with Janine and Robin... helping me to appreciate the simple things in life, such as

- *fresh fruit eaten under a thatched roof hut with chickens eating off of the dirt floor at our feet*

- *creating and sharing poetry as we sat with a group of school children, amid the ruins of an ancient culture long gone*

- *helping children to create and perform plays that showcased their talents, even when they did not realize that they had talents to share... and inviting me to share in your life's work of helping those who needed help... early on, visiting the local prison to bring reading material, blankets, and food to those who were forgotten.*

But, most importantly, Rey, you were my friend... A true, lifelong friend... a fellowship that needs no words; it simply was... We were... We are... We always will be...

Though many years would pass between the time that we traveled together to your parents' home in Taxco, and then a visit in Vermont so many, many years later at Janine's home... those years were like days... time was irrelevant... what more can be said of a true friend, but when two encounter each other after a very long period of time, and the mutual love is evident as though time has not passed. Those are very special friendships... and I thank you for ours. You will forever be in my thoughts and prayers.

Go in peace, my brother; my friend. You have left your mark on this world and it is a better place because of you and all that you have given of yourself to others who needed you. We who were fortunate to be a part of your life are better for having known you. We shall all keep a piece of you in our hearts forever. And, as we strive to help others, we will know that you are looking down upon us and smiling.

Until we meet again,

Jim

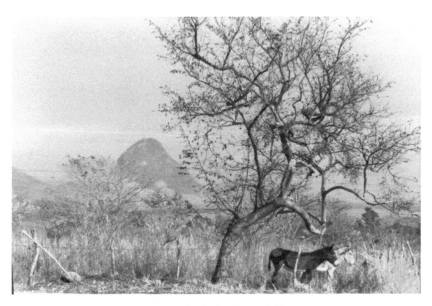

Santa Lucía de La Sierra, Jalisco

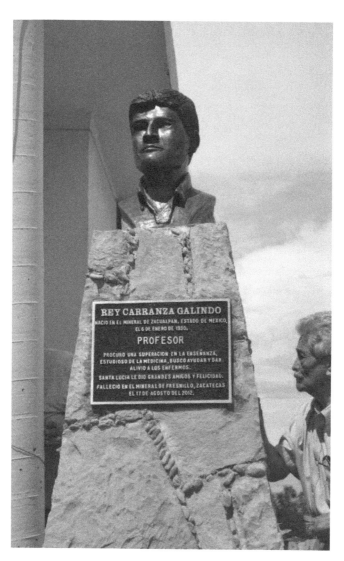

Profe Rey's brother Fernando at statue of Rey Carranza
adjacent to the library Dad built with the villagers.

YouTube: *Rey Carranza "El Professor"*

THE SUFFERING BOWL

When you got so much
You're feeling insane
Come on baby don't hold that pain
Put it in the bowl
The suffering bowl.

Time, lying in the grass
Away you while, alas
Feeling so good you can't help but smile
It's still within reach – the bowl
The suffering bowl.

When you're feeling with another
Sister, friend, Father, Mother
And you can make what's broken whole
Hand-in-hand you'll visit the bowl
The suffering bowl.

It's not a cop-out; It's not a dodge
It's just a place for pain to lodge
While changes swirl about your soul
Why don't you place it in the bowl?
The suffering bowl.

I'll be that bowl for you today.
And tomorrow, perhaps you may
Be the one, the pain to hold,
Perhaps you'll be the bowl
The suffering bowl.

~ Troy Maddux, LMT

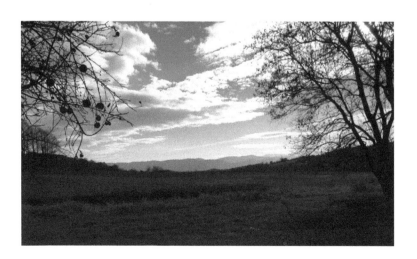

Compassion is someone else's suffering flaring in your own nerves.
Pity is a projection of, a lament for, the self.

~ Christian Wiman

Part Four

THE VALLEY OF UNITY

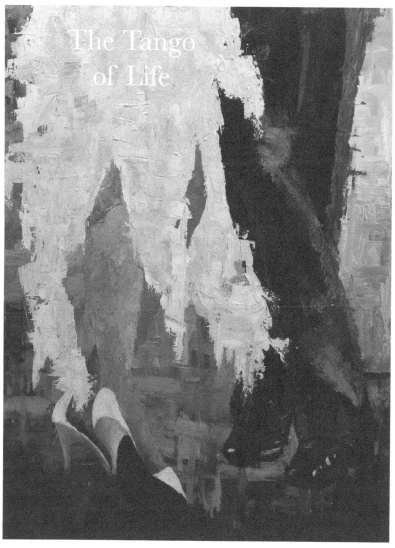

The Tango
of Life

THE DAUGHTER

"Momi, Momi! Look at me Momi!" Momi Angela's eyes stared out the window. They had been closed for most of the month as she wished herself to death.

Her daughter said she knew her mom was ready to go, but that she herself was not ready for her mom to go. *"Don't leave me Momi! Don't leave me!"*

Angela didn't leave her, but she did take her last breath.

"Did she suffocate?" Rosalyn asked afterward. Rosalyn is grown up now... in her 40's? Maybe 30's... I never am good with guessing ages. Rosalyn was 5 and 15 and 35 all at once today. She had so many questions: Was it the morphine? Did she die because she declined oxygen?

Nothing would bring Rosalyn's mother back to earth. Nothing would have stopped her from joining her deceased family when it was over for her here. Not with her husband and son and parents now to welcome her away from her nausea and pain and inability to eat good food. That was her #1 wish when asked: To be able to eat food. But her body would not hold it down, even with sublingual and rectal anti-nausea medications.

"She was about living," her friend said who was bustling taking care of things around the house. *"When she couldn't have that anymore, she was done."* The framed photo on the vanity was of an elegant woman cheek-to-cheek with her husband who spent his life in and out of hospitals. In the photo they looked to be in a fancy dance hall. She had a winning broad smile, and wore the lace dress that her lifeless body now celebrated. A distinct smile lightened her face.

"She is happy," Rosalyn said (Lydia, the steady devoted caregiver, agreed).*"I always irritated her. I would call her every day and she would say, 'Rosalyn, do you have to tell me everything? Can't you save things up, pick the highlights, and call me on the weekend?' But I never could. I was always checking on her. This morning I was folding clothes and I felt I needed to check in on her."*

That was when Rosalyn walked in on her mom's last breaths.

Rosalyn was in tune with her mom. Her mom almost never expressed feelings, she said. *"When my brother died, I never saw her shed a tear. Or talk about it. She kept things from us. She didn't tell me when she was diagnosed with cancer. She didn't tell me when they told her it was terminal. She didn't tell me about Dad or my grandfather's cancer. Even when we had doctor's appointments for ourselves, she would not tell us about it ahead of time. We would arrive at the doctor's and say, 'Mom! At least give us a little time to prepare!' You can see how damaged we are."* She sounded more joking than serious.

"It was like I always needed her, but she never needed me."

Rosalyn had a way of talking about her life story without bitterness. — Either toward her mother or toward herself. She talked a mile a minute… While her mom said almost nothing, even when Momi could, days and weeks ago.

"We weren't allowed to have any sugar. Our parents would take away our Halloween candy. You should see my house now. I have every kind of treat you can imagine. There were never snacks when I was growing up. We had every ingredient you could want. Mom knew how to cook. Really cook. You could find bagels — We would keep those in the freezer. And Mom would make granola; but I never liked granola. My sons can have pop tarts and any snack they want."

Rosalyn laughed and cried at the same time. She and her mom are tiny in physique, pretty, energetic, vivacious. Rosalyn said her mom was part of nearly every organization in town. She cooked for people, attended meetings, took care of details. She knew where every item was in her house, to her last days, *"It is on the left side in the upper drawer, on the top."* She was always right.

Then she put a sign on the door, Asked people to stay away, closed her eyes, Wished herself gone. And she was gone.

THE MOOSE HUNT

The dead mole at the foot of the step
smelled stronger than the last time I was here.
The road to the steps felt more perilous than usual with the leaves off the trees,
making the steep banks on either side of my new work car look steeper still.
Sometimes I couldn't see the road where the deepest drops in elevation were.
The house was between a house and a camp.

Today when I drove up, I wondered where the guns were kept.
No one answered the door this time.
I wouldn't look at the moose head on the wall,
or the bear, or the full-bodied wolf, or the many, many others.
I have tried to not take the dead beasts to heart.
But the consciousness of heavy fur surrounding me,
leaning out toward me in touchable distance, all of us ear to ear, is undeniable.
The loose boards on the porch
that I walked over with my flowing tango slacks on
added to the sense of adventure or peril
as I made my last visit on Friday afternoon,
hoping I might make dancing tonight.

She was gone because she was on her moose hunt.
I had called ahead with no answer, but her medications would be out today.
I needed to fill the pill boxes… So I thought she would be home for that,
even if she was not answering the phone.
(She not answering the phone was not unusual.)

She is a tiny woman in both stature and build
— almost nothing to her.
The animals each seem bigger than she, even the fox.
She walks around that house with a large hole at the side of her neck.

Cancer of the tonsils. She doesn't like to wear the dressing.
So the purulent drainage drips down her neck into her collars.

Her love? Hunting. (Maybe you guessed.)
She sometimes couldn't get to a doctor's office, but she had gone on a moose
hunt. She said it is done by lottery. She got the ticket this time.
Probably for the last time.
I don't know how old she was as a girl when she first won the ticket.
She said she hoped she'd catch her moose on the first day this time around,
because she thought she was going to get tired.
She said they were tracking it ahead of time and knew where it was wandering.

Last week I poured her medications into the day-a-week boxes.
I thought of her all weekend out in the woods with the beautiful sunshine
weather. Now she is not home.
A nursing teacher said to me once,
"When I am working harder than my students are for themselves,
that's when I know to back off."
I don't know how to help her with her medications for the next week.
I won't, I guess.

I will go dancing while she is out getting her moose.

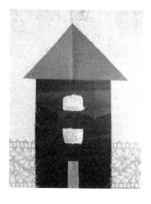

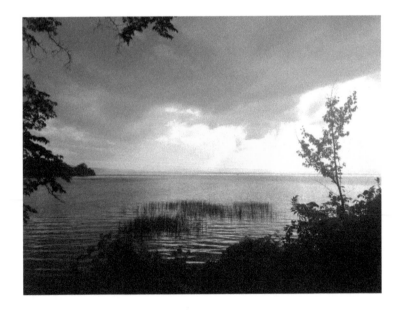

FROM THE SWISS MOUNTAINS

Tomorrow night he goes out with his friends. He will need a neck warmer to cover and keep warm the healing incision from behind his ear, down his neck, plus the side-healing wound from his ear to the front of his face. It won't cover the healing incisions on the front of his face.

It is Wednesday. Sunday was the first day he went out in public, to the Unitarian Church (outside of going to doctors' follow-up appointments, and then a few errands... Farther than his usual stops, in hopes of not coming across anyone he knows). Last night he went to his Italian class.

When he woke up from surgery he didn't know what had happened. He thought it was going to be minor reconstructive surgery he was coming out of, after a cancerous growth had to be removed from his front left cheek. Now he looked in the mirror and didn't know what he was seeing. The wide elastic headband that went from his chin to the top of his head, with a strap over his brow, and a second one behind his head to secure the wider strap, wrapped him unrecognizably. The drain coming out of the side of his neck, with serosanguinous fluid dripping into its drain balloon, did not help coming home to himself.

My job was to clean the wounds, redress them, keep them from getting infected. Nelson hadn't slept for two nights. Sleeping with a protruding drain that was to not get kinked and occluded, plus adjusting to who he was in this new form, made for wakeful hours. He said that once his glass coffee table spontaneously shattered in front of his eyes. He said glass can do that if it hits a particular density sensitivity. *"That's the best way I can describe how I have been feeling,"* he said on the second day, *"Is like shattered glass might feel when impounded upon itself."*

Nelson had a calm, centered, clear, intelligent way of speaking and expressing himself. Everything he said was thought-out. He didn't seem to waste energy or words with nervous distraction. Even irritation was contained when he couldn't swallow from the diverticula in his esophagus. He regurgitated his dinner after finally being able to get a real meal almost down. He made his statements without emotional affect while still expressing deep feeling. He talked about events and days that were profoundly upsetting. His descriptions were both open and contained. I was touched at how he shared his inner world without losing his groundedness in self, without asking for pity or even seeming to ask for understanding. He spoke in the face of truth. He said it because it was there. *"Just fact, no brag,"* is how he might have described it if he was describing.

It was weeks before he left his apartment. Even the Thanksgiving dinner invitations came before he had the strength either physically or psychically to go out of his home-space. And he couldn't take a shower on his own to refresh himself. That was one day it was not hard to forget my productivity numbers at the agency, and help him to take a shower before I redressed his wounds. Then to shave. I combed his beautiful blond-almost orange hair, then put the head-band back on to hold the stitches tight for improved cosmetic healing outcome. The blood on the velcro bands couldn't be changed because we didn't have a replacement and I didn't want to put them on him wet. When I left, I knew that shower had been much better than any anti-depressant pill.

Later his stitches came out, and the drain. A friend who was present, and I, thought he would feel like a new man. *"I would be the one determining that,"* he said without apparent judgment or animosity, just his simple clarity. I immediately acknowledged that he was right about that. I watched him at each of my long wound-cleaning visits. He started to sleep a little better. His eyes became clearer. At first the swelling under his left eye made reading out of his bifocals impossible with that eye. Then the swelling and the eye cleared.

Pockets, or "bulges" as the surgeon called them, became clearly the residual composite of the healing. One elongated section in front of his ear, a contained one on his neck where his shirt collar needs to rest, a third one at the end of the vertical incision down his front cheek. They hadn't been able to pull enough skin over the removed tissue area, so they needed to pull it from farther back, into his neck skin.

The surgeon called it a reverse face lift. The folding and stretching and gathering had left folds. "He can go back to cosmetic surgery in a year," his surgeon said. Whether the shock of this procedure will wear down enough by then for Nelson to consider that remains to be seen. I told him that his expressions and presentation to those around him was not deformed or compromised. I asked him what he saw when he looked in the mirror. He said the bulges. I thought, however, that the folds stood in relatively discreet locations. Maybe I came to see him as himself and couldn't see his scarring anymore. I thought that he could present himself to the world, with dignity, as he looked. I thought his salient qualities of being himself were more powerful than the scars.

He thanked me for helping him find his confidence. For dealing with the whole picture instead of only a "specialized part" that I was trained in, he said. That was an honor. His profession is as a lawyer. But Life had taught him to see life, not a segregated slice from which to make a living. He showed me photos of his landscape views from his home in Switzerland. The far-reaching mountains with the snow, he brings with him in his demeanor.

As he readied to go to his Italian class, I discharged him from home health services. (He was on palliative care, not hospice care). I felt sad to say goodbye. He made me think of my dad: Ageless men. Men who are connected to the world in a more expansive way than the materialized moment of the present.

Doctor's orders to him were to not go out in freezing weather. I took a quick run to Onion River Sports in Montpelier and found him a wide neck warmer, and left it on his doorknob before going home on the dark winter night. I got one for myself too. We needed warmth in a sometimes cold world.

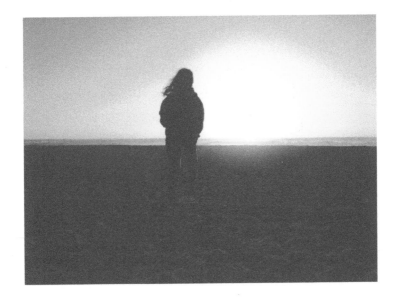

THE PORCH LIGHT

I am so tired tonight that sleeping feels like it wouldn't help. I whole-heartedly wish I had gotten out of work in time to dance tonight. I wish that I could find time to exercise in the work day without compromising basic sleep. I wish that I had time for the special little things of life like polishing the copper on a good pan, or making honey apple crisp, or stopping to take a photo of the round woodpile I often drive by.

When the daughter of the woman with lung cancer and kidney failure, with breast and brain metastases, asked to speak to my supervisor, saying that someone else could come over if I couldn't get there before dark, it all felt too hard. I asked the daughter if coming today before the 4:30 sunset was okay. She wanted an exact time. I knew I couldn't give it. So much in this job derails best-laid plans every hour. I had promised early visits already to two people in town today. Their needs were pressing too. They had already waited more than I wanted them to endure. I told her I could try for 3 pm and call her when I knew the exact time. She said she did not want to be at the bottom of my list.

Part of my being later than I hoped was getting sick yesterday after doing the admission for her mother in their smoke-filled house — my cold that I was trying to ignore, couldn't take it. She didn't know that the late patients are at the top of my list. It is dancing that is at the bottom; and sewing and cooking and having time to take a walk. I miss my friends today. I miss dressing up and feeling pretty and being in shape, innately knowing how to move to a tango song with a partner doing the same.

For my last visit long past dark I didn't even call ahead. It takes her so long to get to the phone that I thought I wouldn't make her go through that effort. I knocked on her unlocked door and she cheerfully said, *"Come in!"* She was at her stove cooking a broth with a bone in it, her walker before her, her green oxygen tubing stretched across the plywood platform that comprised her kitchen floor.

The volunteer had gotten her to a hair appointment the day before. Her hair was cut in a wispy energetic style that made her look like a spry young lady.

"You must have worked long today," Suzanne said. I told her I was sorry it was so late. She said, *"What does it matter?…Where would you like me to sit?"* She acted like interrupting her dinnertime wasn't even happening. She asked me if I had heard the news about the 20 elementary children shot in school in Connecticut. I had not. She said the killer had also killed himself and his mother.

"I am slow moving," she said, inching away from the stove. *"But that I can't change."*

She told me about her day and how the beauty salon had moved around the corner, how she couldn't find it at first, and how nice the lady was. That for Christmas the hairdresser was going to come to her house. She said she was going to otherwise be alone for Christmas, which was fine, that it would be a treat to have her hair done. (It turns out her son was going to be there on Christmas morning and then go see other family.) She said that her last hairdresser would come to her home but that she charged $50. *"This one only charged me $25. I gave her a $5 tip. It was worth it."*

She showed me the painting she was trying to finish for Christmas of a boy and a dog resting their heads on each other. I think it is for the mother of the son in the painting. Behind it was a painting that drew me in, of evergreens almost framing the composition, and an orange sky behind. It felt real and alive without sentimentalism or clichés. I commented on it. She said she had just thought of that picture yesterday. And that she wants to soften it and give it the feeling of a fog. She asked me if I had to undo the closely criss-crossed laces on the tall boots I was wearing to get my boots off. I told her to close her eyes. She did. I unzipped the hidden side zipper on my boots, without touching the laces, and had them off in a minute. When she opened her eyes she said, *"There's a zipper."* We laughed. Her home, her food on the stove cooking, her cheerfulness and engagement after being one of the ten admissions I took into hospice last week, her frank attention and straightforward connection, shone in her with a very special beauty to me tonight: Her capacity to engage in problem-solving to make her life in her small home work for her in small ways, her capacity to accept help with grace, her love for her son who both helps her and respects her autonomy. The lights in her windows with the porch light on even if she was not expecting me… It all touched my heart, just when I thought I could not do one more visit, with my friends visiting and dancing to music far away. Suzanne was not far away. For the moment I was happy sitting in a chair she cleared off for me and looking into her lovely face, listening to her. For the moment everything was okay.

Even if I had cried a lot today missing my father and the common struggles he had in his similar work. Cried that I so rarely see my friends any more. Cried that my body is so tired and that I haven't been able to take good care of it. it. Cried because the local grocery store closed the door in front of me even if it wasn't their closing time of 8pm yet, and I couldn't buy the apples I wanted for my apple crisp — they used to be a small local Vermont grocery store before the chain took it over.

Despite all, I had been able to give a hug to the woman who had yelled at me earlier, as she was crying with her mom in the smoky house.

With a porch light at the end of the day, and having found a way to help a distraught family, I know I can do this.

*"Sometimes the best answer to exhaustion is not rest,
but rather wholeheartedness."*

~ Brother David Steindl-Rast, as quoted by David Whyte

THE TASTE OF LIFE

"I am sorry the stethoscope is so cold." Garth rolled his eyes. *"After what I have been through, and you think your stethoscope is going to bother me?"* "Well, sometimes one more thing can really bother when you've gone through what you have."

"You know, I am careful now at what I let bother me. There's not a lot that gets to me now. I've got my kids. They're good to me. I care about them. I don't worry about a lot of other stuff any more. It gives you a different perspective to see the end stare you in the face. I didn't know if I was going to make it this far. Now I am going to enjoy it. People may think I am crazy, the way I talk, but I don't care what people think any more. I say what I have to say."

That morning he had overflowed many gallons of perfected maple syrup onto the shop floor. He ran a maple syrup business in his garage. We sat next to the shiny boiler. The floor was polished from the mopping-up. I had bought a gallon (of the not-spilled stuff) to refill my low supply at home — If it weren't for maple syrup, I think I would live out West.

He sat comfortably in his chair. He was the guy who didn't want a visiting nurse. But today we felt like friends. Neighbors. Vermonters. He chatted about his life while doing the discharge paperwork, now that he was going to take care of himself after the healing of his successful surgery at round-two of kidney cancer.

"I learned to use my head instead of my fist from an early age. Once I was sitting at a bar with a guy twice my size. I was pushing his buttons. He said he'd knock me one if I didn't let up. I didn't let up. He punched me in the chin. I looked right at him and said, 'If you hit me again, and I know about it, you're going to piss me off.' He looked at me in surprise, and then started to laugh. We didn't give each other any trouble after that. I never drank much but I used to like a beer in the afternoon. He bought me my beer that day."

"Then there was a guy who was pushing my buttons. He asked me to step outside. The bar was quiet... Seeing what would happen. I told him it was cold outside. 'You're a loser,' he said. The only thing I have lost tonight is my respect for you. As a local business man, you should be ashamed of yourself, the way you are acting.' He left the bar soon after that. There was nothing left for him to fight.

"When a neighbor kid came and jumped on the trunk of my son's new Volvo, my son started yelling, 'get off my car!' I went over to the boy and said, 'You know you're going to have to pay for that.' The boy said, 'Oh yeah? Who says?' 'I say for now. Or it can be someone else if you want.'

You can do a lot more with your brain than your body. And it doesn't hurt as much," Garth said. I asked him if his son was good at that kind of tactic. "Oh, yeah. He's better. I wouldn't be alive today if it weren't for my kids," he reminisced.

His son drove up in his Volvo. His daughter was at work. The home was small, comfortable, and did what a home needs to do. It was enough.

Garth's life was enough for him.

Figuring out how to pay for the addition to the boiler that would protect the overflows and wastes of syrup was also part of his world. His warmth, his love for his son and daughter who lived there too, their taking over his business when he no longer will be able to, his finding the energy to do the work now, is what he cares about.

The flavor in the air from the from the boiler aromatics, lingered. Life is sweet when we can taste it.

WHEN IT'S TIME
FOR PALLIATIVE CARE

"It's not over till it's over and I was hoping it was over;
It's one foot forward and two feet back, like whistling in the wind. Is it worth it?
We're older and we manage, but don't talk about quality of life
because we don't have it; it's non-existent.
Here are two independent people, dependent. My zip is zapped.
Taking care of things around the house takes all I've got."

I asked him if there is anything he and his wife look forward to.

"Being together."
He was the guy who had said one day, winking at his wife,
"I used to get out of breath…" he hesitated, glancing at his wife
to see if she wanted to stop him; she was smiling,
"I used to get out of breath when she would come in topless to take care of my
feet." Breathing came hard for him with his emphysema.

"It would be nice to be holding hands in bed."

He has been sleeping in the recliner for better mobility,
so I started talking about the option of sleeping in the bed with alterations
that would enable him to be able to get out from the bed shared with her,
which was the issue for not sleeping in his bed at night.

"That is not what I was talking about. I am talking about the end.
I'd like to take something [to die], but we can't do that.
I will probably go first. I am younger than she is.
But neither of us wants to go first and leave the other behind."

They are now both my patients, after she fell and fractured her vertebrae.

"The warmer weather is something to look forward to, if we can get out.
We used to go on long drives together. I know those days are over.
It is a windy road with a lot of detours.
I am looking forward to what Dr. Zahm says, and then the cardiologist in March.
But what then?
It's like Zahm and I are going steady, and I don't like it.
I don't even like doctors and hospitals.
I fought all my life to not have to deal with that, now I have no choice.

I bow to the professionals — Dr. Zahm is a good doctor — don't get me wrong.
But my zip is zapped.

Enough, I say; Enough."

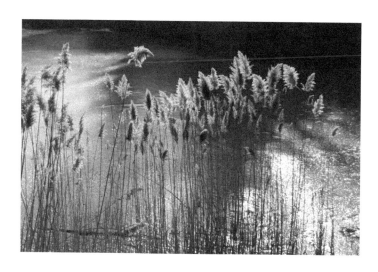

DROPLETS OFF THE EVES

Paul sat in his wheelchair, a man with the energy of a 40-year-old, actually a decade older than that. Four months ago he was walking around his house doing his carpentry. He decided to have surgery for a severely degenerated vertebral disc. His pain was frustratingly interfering with his work. He came out of the surgery without sensation below the waist.

Last week he seriously considered killing himself. He said he did not want to put his wife and family through what they do for him. He and his family already overcame two invasions of advanced cancer since 2001. First lymphoma, then cancer in the spleen. But it was talking about suicide that upset his wife most, she said.

He said it took him twenty-five years to take out of his head the vision of his dying emaciated mother, whom he took care of. That was in the days before hospice was well developed and accessible. Today he can see her at peace. But he could not for a long time.

His home is extraordinarily beautiful, created by their own hands. He and his family are even more beautiful. He said that he is Jewish but, that with the death of his mother, he lost his faith. He looked confused, and said he was.

He has exceptionally clear eyes. There is an intelligence and a calm in their deep brown color — a resilience that does not fit the talk of suicide at a young age.

He said his family and friends had a healing circle on top of the hill for him when he came back from chemotherapy one year. He pointed up a steep rise directly outside his kitchen window. The snow covered the ground in a thin layer. The tree trunks looked dispersed as if perfectly planned. The sun and its rays streaked onto us through the trees. The drips from the spring day fell from the eves in musical sounds.

He went to rehab — the best one in Vermont. With leg braces he can now move around his house with a walker. He thinks he has enough movement in his left foot to be able to drive again. He needs a urinary catheter — that feels like a leash, he said. Tying himself to a tube feels like it pulls him farther from his beautiful, active and devoted wife.

The pain in his bladder spreads to his intestines. He will not take narcotics for fear of the side effect of constipation — even if bowel medications could take care of that problem. But it might not help the cramping anyway. He is taking neuropathic medications for severe nerve pain… not high enough doses… Gabapentin does not hurt the liver. His liver is struggling: Hepatitis C, cirrhosis… Gradual increased Gabapentin levels, up to 900mg three times a day (his nerve pain medicine) gave him the relief he needed from constant unbearable shooting pain. He wants to lighten the load on his liver, as many medications filter through the liver… Does he need Lactulose to help prevent ammonia toxicity and mental status changes and to help with the bowels? Maybe it is too early for that… We'll check the liver tests… Check the methadone level… We finessed the details and managed the pain that before was finding him doubled up when receiving visitors and professionals.

A man with dignity, an active love life, intellectually developed, socially connected, now spending most of his time in the bathroom trying to relieve unbearable cramping that does not let up. Sleep is all he longs for sometimes, and even that can be rare.

I asked him about his wishes. He said that if he got his life back, that he would want to return to nursing. He used to work for the agency I work in now. With his failing liver that may be a far stretch. Maybe he can take the hospice volunteer training.

Day one on a new path: We talked about what he wanted to embrace in each new day and what to let go of. Today a catheter is a start — at least until we can isolate the bladder spasms from a full bladder. Sitting in the sunshine with him for three hours, we unraveled the tangles… Inviting his friend Kateyn over to practice guitar is his immediate wish. Tonight music is the call.

• • •

Crying in the car at the end of the day, with my father's loss never far, I texted Michael for consolation.

"U live a beautiful and a hard life,"

he texted back to me, in his own stressful day from which he has not had a day off all year,

"and the two are inextricable."

I could hear the droplets from the eaves in this fragile and resilient world.

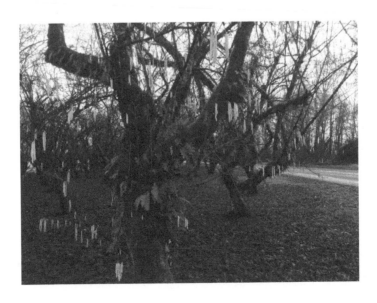

THE NEW YORK TIMES REPORTER

I let the dog out of the apartment. He barked his high incessant bark as if he did not know me. Cindy asked me to let him out when I stopped by to pick up the extra supplies that Cameron no longer needed. Pepe ran across the driveway into the soft fur dog bed that he had greeted me in since December 12th in Cameron's apartment. The hospital bed was still there. It looked like it feels when you go back to a childhood home and you wonder where the magic went. And this was one day later, not after decades of adulthood.

The day-before-yesterday, Cameron was in that bed where it took 40mg of morphine to keep away the pain from the bone metastases of his prostate cancer. A lot of his body had been numb during the months of the progression of the cancer, but now at the end it rammed him.

Thank goodness for Amy, a PCA who came to spend the night so that the son, who could hardly stand from exhaustion, could get some sleep — not just because she let Adam sleep, but because Cameron could only tell her, and not us, that he was hurting. She was a stranger. Her clear communication, bright young face, and simplicity of questions, freed Cameron to speak of his symptoms. To the son and family, and me and David my colleague, Cameron held back from saying how much he hurt because he was close to us.

At 10:30 pm Cameron was still able to speak. He was getting morphine anyway, because I knew he understated pain, but he continually said, *"no"* he was not hurting, and even, *"no I am fine."* His thrashing in the bed spoke differently. I increased the MSIR (Morphne instant release), and weighed constantly the balance of terminal agitation (which the Olanzapaine had helped) and the pain.

When the verbal communication is broken down, what symptom to treat strongest, is where the art of hospice comes in. Knowledge of the patient's past symptoms up to now is most of the battle won, the non-verbal symptoms almost the other half, as in the brow that shows tension to the end, when the mouth no longer can. The rest is the sign that is given by grace from one source or another, along with the assumption that it is always to some degree both pain and terminal upset. Each to what degree for treatment is the question.

If Cameron had not been opening his eyes, giving me eye contact and saying repeatedly over the hours, while thrashing, that he was not hurting, I would have increased the morphine (within the doctor's order-range in place) until he became restful, knowing full-well that bone pain is intense. Increasing the morphine to high doses while he insisted he was not hurting, nor showed signs of difficulty breathing, is not good nursing practice. Was all this fear and restlessness?

Just as I was thinking that I had to be aggressive about either the agitation or the pain, but which one? or both? Amy came in and Cameron spoke the words of grace to the puzzle: *"My back is hurting."* So between that time and 2am, Amy was the communicator, I was the hospice nurse, and we watched his pain relieved with each added dose of increased morphine. Forty milligram doses became his relief dose. Scheduling it for every four hours to keep ahead of the pain did the trick. He still needed two extra doses before I came back the next day at noon. He was at peace with that and the Olanzapine.

"I am not afraid of dying," he had said to me with perfect clarity and consciousness on one of my first meetings with him, *"I am afraid of what comes between here and there."* I got it. I talked to him about hospice. I told him that this piece was our job. He said he knew a lot about it from hospice helping him take care of his wife who died of parkinsons under his care in 2010. And their 53-year-old daughter had died in 2007, also of cancer.

He said he could handle the end. I told him I would manage the arrangements between. How to do that during the time he was on hospice, with both his understatement of symptoms and also his living "alone", took some consciousness and patience to figure out. He didn't accept nursing aide help for baths until the last days of his life. He handled his personal care up to that point. On another visit we talked about using Vermont Respite House as a back-up if his care needs couldn't be handled at home. The unfolding was unpredictable; we took one day at a time.

The biggest challenge in those four months, from day one, was reading him outside of the man who did not want to bother people. When his granddaughter and I stood on either side of his dead body while his son had gone out to get sandwiches, she said that he encouraged people to do their thing — that he didn't need or like people hovering. This granddaughter is the daughter of Cameron's daughter who had died in 2007, at the age of 53.

Cameron spoke of his joy in watching his son Adam handle the huge snowstorms with the snow plows from Adam's business. That is Cameron's son's job for local ski businesses. *"I have known what he does, but watching him with his equipment, his foresight of what is needed, his efficiency and energy and management of the team, and how well he does it, has been really great. I am glad I have been able to see that."* Cameron spoke of the holiday catering business run by his daughter-in-law Cindy in which she worked with the same expertise, purpose, and engagement.

His apartment across from their house was perfect. He felt he could be less of a burden, but still close to family. They led their lives and made him his meals and looked after his needs, he led his life.

Dinnertime was their time together in his apartment. Appetite was joyously something he did not lose until the very last days. The only thing he came up with on a "bucket list" was special food items. He got repetitions on those requests, like the Crème Brûlée both Cindy and I made him in the same week. It is all we could give him that he directly asked for.

He said he had done his life. He contemplated my question of whether he wanted in his long quiet days to give an oral history of his interesting life. He thought about it. Then was very clear that he did not need to do that. I asked him if his family knew the stories of his full life as a New York Times reporter and the intrigue of his history. *"Oh yes,"* he said.

He had been active and purposeful in his life — engaged physically and intellectually. Even when he took care of his wife, he had active and serious purpose. Now what? His fatigue was too great to do more than finish his taxes for 2012 so he would not leave that for his son (he completed that), and send out his Christmas cards and gifts when that season came in 2012 (he completed that), and then die as soon as possible. This was how he wished it.

He read up on assisted suicide. It was not legal in Vermont at that time. He knew that.

He had an electronic book to read that his family gave him for Christmas. He finished reading it. He showed me about the augmenting rhythm of crossword puzzles: How there is that point of critical mass after which the connections between the words and the integration of his mind and the mind of the author, rolls into a rhythm where the words complete themselves. He kept up on the news.

He taught me about the chapel's process of electing a new Pope, and the smoke-sign from the cardinals with resolution. He had his favorite interviewer whom he kept up on with the introductions to interesting people.

One day he talked about the days the press got a momentous piece of news.

"It made us see how all the preparation and training and organization with staff was worth it. It was in those times that everything we worked for came together and made sense. People let go their 'meshugeh' from slower days and it was amazing to watch the efficiency and skill and coming together of all of us." His face lit up as he talked as if seeing it happen before him — as if we were in the newsroom together. People working in sync: *"There is nothing like it,"* he said.

He said that he accepted a position at one point to oversee 150 of the staff, but when they hired someone under him to do his old job, he felt he lost control of the judgment calls that gave the work meaning and expertise. He didn't like answering to other people's choices and feeling a step away from implementing those choices to his personal standards, he said.

He said it was a great epoch to have been involved in the newspaper business. He started with the manual printers, implemented the computer systems himself, and thrived on the best of the new system before its current challenges.

He was not a big talker, as I have intimated. When he spoke it was memorable. There was a vague feeling, every time I was coming up his driveway, that we would have nothing to talk about. That he would not tell me how he was feeling, and that I would have nothing to do there. Just like when I sat down to write this story, it felt like I wouldn't have anything to write, despite my full heart. That was never how it panned out.

I worked at not filling silence with chatter. It was okay to be quiet, as when I filled the syringes with the medication for him to have easy access (mostly the Lorazepam so he could calm his understated restlessness). The visits were usually short, but we talked about the basics, worked at keeping the stability and treating the exacerbations. When I was lucky, I would get gems of his thoughts.

He would have once, twice, or three times a week tough days. Days when all he could do was stay in bed due to pain. Usually my visits would miss these days. He had the oral syringes (without needles) with medication combos in the house to treat them, along with the vicodin pills he took at the time.

One day when I arrived on his bad day, he was sobbing. *"Why can't I just die?"* he said. Then apologized for saying that. I asked him why he was sorry. He said because it upsets people to hear that. I told him that I wanted him to speak his mind. That it helped me help him. That day was the only day he accepted a back rub from me. He was comfortable when I left his doors. Until his next episode.

From February 21st to March 19th he had clear days. No bad ones. For him, it was a long stretch. On one visit during this time, his chronic low grade fever was gone, his irregular, rapid heartbeat was even and slowed down, he had been weeks without a 'bad day'. *"I am going to ask them to get me my car back."* he said with a smile.

When his granddaughter and I stood in front of each other on either side of his bed, and he taking his last breaths, she called Adam on her cell. She put the phone to her grandfather's ear and Adam told his dad how much he loved him. Cameron took an extended breath, his last one.

"You planned that," Emily said to her grandfather: To go when Adam was out getting sandwiches. He planned it to die with his son's love in his ear, and also to not burden his son with his passing — because they are so close. Emily said it was completely in line with Cameron's needs for privacy and not being a burden. *"He used to say, 'you go do your thing.'"* She said her mom did the same. She said her mom had said to her, *"It is time for you to go now."* She said she had taken time off and was staying with her mom to take care of her. *"'Okay',* Emily told her. *'If that is the way you want it.'"* Her mom died within days. Emily said she got it. She understood that her mother needed this privacy.

Emily cried and talked about the loss of her mother and her own fear of death. I asked her if seeing her grandfather take his last breath made the fear more or less. She said that she saw that he didn't struggle. She talked of her dreams of her mother.

When we talked about new dreams in contrast to memory dreams with people who are dead, and that the new dreams are said to be visits from your loved one coming back to be with you, she said, *"I will ride with that."*

After Adam came back with his face swollen from days of sleeplessness and tears, they stepped out for me to clean the body. I was alone for the job with the still flaccid cooling corpse, and the pooling of his blood under the surface of the backside of his skin. I was used to doing this part alone, but tonight I texted David, my now nursing partner in the valley, to see if he was close by to help me (he lives five minutes away), but he was still in Boston on a trip. I was trying hard to swallow down crying. My boss called right then and thanked me for the work I had done with the family. Her backing helped.

On my drive back to the satellite office, I gobbled down the huge vegetarian sandwich with delicious crispy bread that Adam had brought back for me. I was hungry after the long hours of holding presence with this family. I thanked the universe for it being my last visit for the day. When my boss called for an emergency catheter insertion, I told myself it was because of my desperate back-log of charting that I asked her to find someone else. But it was more than that. I drove home with deep crying inside me. I did not want to cry out loud more than I had already since the last death of a few days ago.

I thought of the night before, getting home at 3am, after getting Cameron comfortable. Two pairs of deer stood in the field before our home, under a burgeoning half moon, amidst lengthy clouds lit with stark borders from the dark background. The night felt pregnant. I didn't know for what. I didn't know that tomorrow at 1:30pm Cameron would take his last breath under the care of his granddaughter. That he would close his life as he asked to.

Pepe, asleep in his bed next to the empty hospital bed, took in the stroking. I backed down the steep dirt driveway that only once in that winter kept my car from making it up. Adam was away on his vacation. His dad wanted him to go. Cameron died the day before the flight, making way. *"You go do your thing,"* Cameron said. His family shared their personal destinies and fulfillments. There was no burden.

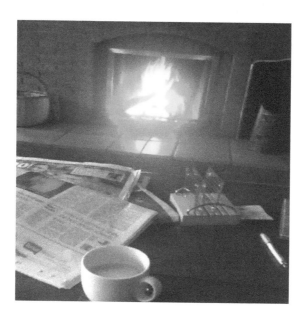

IN THE GARDEN

There was a young girl, Bonnie, who lived with her mother and grandmother.
Her mother liked the gardens at their home, and spent a lot of time there.
Her grandmother was not allowed to go get Mother from the gardens.
That was Mother's space.
So she sent Bonnie instead (Bonnie was allowed).

It is many years later. Now it is Bonnie, remembering those days,
as she is taking care of her husband's aunt Veronica.
Now it is Bonnie who has found herself in the gardens, asking to not be called.
"I understand my mother now."

Aunt Veronica, the 99-year-old woman now in Bonnie's care, lived with angst,
Bonnie says with affection and acceptance.
"She's angry. She fought life and now she is fighting death."
I don't know the details about the way Veronica lived and struggled,
nor had time to catch up on that now.
Veronica lay thrashing in bed unresponsive to our words or interventions.
She was not finding relief
in the multiple avenues of comfort intervention implemented.
It was not physical pain; she had never had pain issues.
Hour past hour dragged by without peace.
Veronica was crying out and moaning in deep agony with terminal agitation.
It was likely that her failing liver
was not allowing the medication to be absorbed.

The next step was phenobarbital, a barbiturate and powerful sedative,
since the less extreme medications were ineffective,
even at high and frequent doses.
It was 8pm and our system to get this medication after hours
was yet to be set up.

The family and she had been adamant
that they did not want her to go to an inpatient unit or the hospital.

There is nothing in this work more depleting than being unsuccessful hour
after hour in giving relief and comfort. It doesn't happen often.
(It didn't help that this was the night I was supposed to get a half day off,
the night I save to see my daughter.
I had already called Anya and told her I couldn't be there.)
I love my work, but I do not like to leave my family unattended.
I had arrived at 3pm to the remote home near the cascading brook
with the rough waters that flowed below the steep decline off the dirt road.
It was 9pm now. I was leaving with maybe 50% success in calming Veronica.
My hope and expectation was that the medications would catch up with her.

They did, I heard later, after a few more hours and more medications
from the detailed written instructions left.
Her last days after that difficult night were quiet.
She did not end up needing or using the phenobarbital we got the next day.

Bonnie and her husband were getting on in years themselves.
Those long stressful hours and loss of sleep
were a bit more than their bodies knew how to tolerate,
and a lot more than they thought they were getting into.
(It took me days, myself, to recuperate.)

Veronica died on Bonnie's birthday,
seven years to date of the day she moved in.
Bonnie said she can visit her in her gardens now.
Bonnie and her husband
said that for a while they were going to sleep when they were tired
and eat when they were hungry, and not much else.
A novel plan.

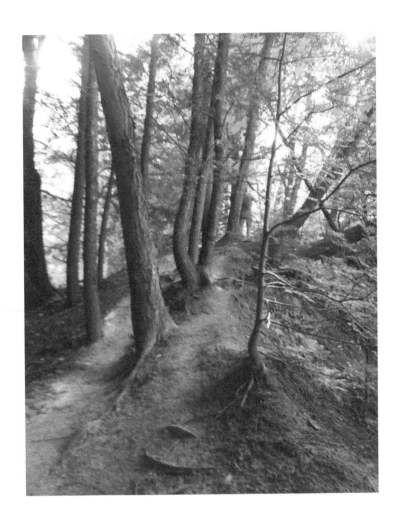

THE ROAD TO TINKHAMTOWN
by Corey Ford

The road was long, but he knew where he was going. He would follow the old road through the swamp and up over the ridge and down to a deep ravine, and cross the sagging timbers of the bridge, and on the other side would be the place called Tinkhamtown. He was going back to Tinkhamtown.

He walked slowly, for his legs were dragging, and he had not been walking for a long time. He had not walked for almost a year, and his flanks had shriveled and wasted away from lying in bed so long; he could fit his fingers around his thigh. Doc. Towle had said he would never walk again, but that was Doc for you, always on the pessimistic side. Why, here he was walking quite easily, once he had started. The strength was coming back into his legs, and he did not have to stop for breath so often. He tried jogging a few steps, just to show he could, but he slowed again because he had a long way to go.

It was hard to make out the old road, choked with young alders and drifted over with matted leaves, and he shut his eyes so he could see it better. He could always see it whenever he shut his eyes. Yes, here was the beaver dam on the right, just as he remembered it, and the flooded stretch where he had to wade, picking his way from hummock to hummock while the dog splashed unconcernedly in front of him. The water had been over his boot tops in one place, and sure enough as he waded it now, his left boot filled with water again, the same warm, squidgy feeling. Everything was the way it had been that afternoon. Nothing had changed. Here was the blow down across the road that he had clambered over and here on a knoll was the clump of thorn apples where Cider had put up a grouse — he remembered the sudden road as the grouse thundered out, and the easy shot that he missed — they had not taken time to go after it. Cider had wanted to look for it, but he had whistled him back. They were looking for Tinkhamtown.

Everything was the way he remembered. There was a fork in the road, and he halted and felt in the pocket of his hunting coat and took out the map he had drawn twenty years ago. He had copied it from a chart he found in the Town Hall, rolled up in a cardboard cylinder covered with dust. He used to study the old survey charts; sometimes they showed where a farming community had flourished once, and around the abandoned pastures and under the apple trees, grown up to pine, the grouse would be feeding undisturbed. Some of his best grouse-covers had been located that way. The chart had crackled with age as he unrolled it; the date was 1847. It was the sector between Kearsarge and Cardigan Mountains, a wasteland of slash and second-growth timber without habitation today, but evidently it had supported a number of families before the Civil War. A road was marked on the map, dotted with X's for homesteads and the names of the owners were lettered beside them: Nason, J. Tinkham, Libbey, Allard, R. Tinkham. Half the names were Tinkham. In the center of the map — the paper was so yellow he could barely make it out — was the word Tinkhamtown.

He copied the chart carefully, noting where the road turned off at the base of Kearsage and ran north and then northeast and crossed a brook that was not even named on the chart; and early the next morning he and Cider had set out together to find the place. They could not drive very far in the jeep, because washouts had gutted the roadbed and laid bare the ledges and boulders, like a streambed. He had stuffed the sketch in his hunting-coat pocket, and hung his shotgun over his forearm and started walking, the old setter trotting ahead of him, with the bell on his collar tinkling. It was an old-fashioned sleighbell, and it had a thin silvery note that echoed through the woods like peepers in the spring; he could follow the sound in the thickest cover, and when it stopped, he would go to where he heard it last and Cider would be on point. After Cider's death, he had put the bell away. He'd never had another dog.

It was silent in the woods without the bell, and the way was longer than he remembered. He should have come to the big hill by now. Maybe he'd taken the wrong turn back at the fork. He thrust a hand into his hunting-coat; the sketch he had drawn was still in the pocket. He sat down on a flat rock to get his bearings, and then he realized, with a surge of excitement, that he had stopped for lunch on this very rock ten years ago. Here was the waxed paper from his sandwich, tucked in a crevice, and here was the hollow in the leaves where Cider had stretched out beside him, the dog's soft muzzle flattened on his thighs. He looked up, and through the trees he could see the hill.

He rose and started walking again, carrying his shotgun. He had left the gun standing in its rack in the kitchen, when he had been taken to the state hospital, but now it was hooked over his arm by the trigger guard; he could feel the solid heft of it. The woods were more dense as he climbed, but here and there a shaft of sunlight slanted through the trees. "And the forests ancient as the hills," he thought, "enfolding sunny spots of greenery." Funny that should come back to him now; he hadn't read it since he was a boy. Other things were coming back to him, the smell of the dank leaves and the sweet fern and frosted apples, the sharp contrast of sun and the cold November shade, the stillness before snow. He walked faster, feeling the excitement swell within him.

He paused on the crest of the hill, straining his ears for the faint mutter of the stream below him, but he could not hear it because of the voices. He wished they would stop talking, so he could hear the stream. Someone was saying his name over and over. Someone said, "What is it, Frank?" and he opened his eyes. Doc Towle was standing at the foot of the bed, whispering to the new nurse, Mrs. Simmons or something; she'd only been here a few days, but Doc thought it would take some of the burden off his wife. He turned his head on the pillow, and looked up at his wife's face, bent over him. "What did you say, Frank?" she asked, and her face was worried. Why, there was nothing to be worried about. He wanted to tell her where he was going, but when he moved his lips no sound came. "What?" she asked, bending her head lower. "I don't hear you." He couldn't make the words any clearer, and she straightened and said to Doc Towle: "It sounded something like Tinkhamtown."

"Tinkhamtown?" Doc shook his head. "Never heard him mention any place by that name."

He smiled to himself. Of course he'd never mentioned it to Doc. There are some things you don't mention even to an old hunting companion like Doc. Things like a secret grouse cover you didn't mention to anyone, not even to as close a friend as Doc was. No, he and Cider were the only ones who knew. They had found it together, that long ago afternoon, and it was their secret. "This is our secret cover," he had told Cider that afternoon, as he lay sprawled under the tree with the grouse beside him and the dog's muzzle flattened on his thigh. "Just you and me." He had never told anybody else about Tinkhamtown, and he had never gone back after Cider died.

He had walked all that morning, stopping now and then to study the map and take his bearings from the sun, and the road had led them down a long hill and at the bottom was the brook he had seen on the chart, a deep ravine spanned by a wooden bridge. Cider had trotted across the bridge, and he had followed more cautiously, avoiding the loose planks and walking the solid struts with his shotgun held out to balance himself; and that was how he found Tinkhamtown.

On the other side of the brook was a clearing, he remembered, and the remains of a stone wall, and a cellar-hole where a farmhouse had stood. Cider had moved in a long cast around the edge of the clearing, his bell tinkling faintly, and he had paused a moment beside the foundations, wondering about the people who had lived here a century ago. Had they ever come back to Tinkhamtown? And then suddenly, the bell had stopped, and he had hurried across the clearing. An apple tree was growing in a corner of the stone wall, and under the tree Cider had halted at point. He could see it all now: the warm October sunlight, the ground strewn with freshly-pecked apples, the dog standing immobile with one foreleg drawn up, his back level and his tail a white plume. Only his flanks quivered a little, and a string of slobber dangled from his jowls. "Steady, boy," he murmured as he moved up behind him, "I'm coming."

"Better let him rest," he head Doc tell his wife. It was funny to hear them talking, and not be able to make them hear him. "Call me if there's any change."

The old road lay ahead of him, dappled with sunshine. He could smell the dank leaves, and feel the chill of the shadows under the hemlocks; it was more real than the pain in his legs. Sometimes it was hard to tell what was real and what was something he remembered. Sometimes at night he would hear Cider panting on the floor beside his bed, his toenails scratching as he chased a bird in a dream, but when the nurse turned on the light the room would be empty. And then when it was dark he would hear the panting and scratching again.

Once he asked Doc point blank about his legs. "Will they ever get better?" He and Doc had grown up in town together; they knew each other too well to lie. Doc had shifted his big frame in the chair beside the bed, and got out his pipe and fumbled with it, and looked at him. "No, I'm afraid not," he replied slowly, "I'm afraid there's nothing to do." Nothing to do but lie here and wait till it's over. Nothing to do but lie here like this, and be waited on, and be a burden to everybody. He had a little insurance, and his son in California sent what he could to help, but now with the added expense of a nurse and all… "Tell me, Doc," he whispered, for his voice wasn't as strong these days, "what happens when it's over?" And Doc put away the needle and fumbled with the catch of his black bag and said he supposed that you went on to someplace else called the Hereafter. But he shook his head; he always argued with Doc. "No," he told him, "it isn't someplace else. It's someplace you've been where you want to be again, someplace you were happiest." Doc didn't understand, and he couldn't explain it any better. He knew what he meant, but the shot was taking effect and he was tired. The pain had been worse lately, and Doc had started giving him shots with a needle so he could sleep. But he didn't really sleep, because the memories kept coming back to him, or maybe he kept going back to the memories.

He paused on the crest of the hill, straining his ears for the faint mutter of the stream below him, but he could not hear it because of the voices. He wished they would stop talking, so he could hear the stream. Someone was saying his name over and over. They had come to the stream – he shut his eyes so he could see it again — and Cider had trotted across the bridge. He had followed more cautiously, avoiding the loose planks and walking on a beam, with his shotgun held out to balance himself. On the other side the road rose sharply to a level clearing and he paused beside the split-stone foundation of a house. The fallen timbers were rotting under a tangle of briars and burdock, and in the empty cellar hole the cottonwoods grew higher than the house had been. His toe encountered a broken china cup and the rusted rims of a wagon wheel buried in the grass.

Beside the granite doorsill was a lilac bush planted by the woman of the family to bring a touch of beauty to their home. Perhaps her husband had chided her for wasting time on such useless things, with as much work to be done. But all the work had come to nothing. The fruits of their work had disappeared, and still the lilac bloomed each spring, defying the encroaching forest, as thought to prove that beauty is the only thing that lasts.

On the other side of the clearing were the sills of the barn, and behind it a crumbling stone wall around the orchard. He thought of the men sweating to clear the fields and pile the rocks into walls to hold their cattle. Why had they gone away from Tinkhamtown, leaving their walls to crumble and their buildings to collapse under the January snows? Had they ever come back to Tinkhamtown? Or were they still here, watching him unseen, living in a past that was more real than the present. He stumbled over a block of granite, hidden by briars, part of the sill of the old barn. Once it had been a tight barn, warm with cattle steaming in their stalls and sweet with the barn odor of manure and hay and leather harness. It seemed as though it was more real to him than the bare foundation and the empty space about them. Doc used to argue that what's over is over, but he would insist Doc was wrong. Everything is the way it was, he'd tell Doc. The present always changes, but the past is always the way it was. You leave it, and go to the present, but it is still there, waiting for you to come back to it.

He had been so wrapped up in his thoughts that he had not realized Cider's bell had stopped. He hurried across the clearing, holding his gun ready. In a corner of the stone wall an ancient apple tree had covered the ground with red fruit, and beneath it Cider was standing motionless. The white fan of his tail was lifted a little, his neck stretched forward, and one foreleg was cocked. His flanks were trembling, and a thin skein of drool hung from his jowls. The dog did not move as he approached, but he could see the brown eyes roll back until their whites showed, waiting for him. His throat grew tight, the way it always did when Cider was on point, and he swallowed hard. "Steady, boy," he whispered, "I'm coming."

He opened his eyes. His wife was standing beside his bed and his son was standing near her. He looked at his son. Why had he come all the way from

California, he worried? He tried to speak, but there was no sound. "I think his lips moved just now. He's trying to whisper something," his wife's voice said. "I don't think he knows you," his wife said to his son. Maybe he didn't know him. Never had, really. He had never been close to his wife or his son. He did not open his eyes, because he was watching for the grouse to fly as he walked past Cider, but he knew Doc. Towle was looking at him. "He's sleeping," Doc said after a moment. Maybe you better get some sleep yourself. A chair creaked, and he heard Doc's heavy footsteps cross the room. "Call me if there's any change," Doc said, and closed the door, and in the silence he could hear his wife sobbing beside him, her dress rustling regularly as she breathed. How could he tell her he wouldn't be alone? But he wasn't alone, not with Cider. He had the old dog curled on the floor by the stove, his claws scratching the linoleum as he chased a bird in a dream. He wasn't alone when he heard that. They were always together. There was a closeness between them that he did not feel for anyone else, his wife, his son, or even Doc. They could talk without words, and they could always find each other in the woods. He was lost without him. Cider was the kindest person he had ever known.

They never hunted together after Tinkhamtown. Cider had acted tired, walking back to the car that afternoon, and several times he sat down on the trail, panting hard. He had to carry him in his arms the last hundred yards to the jeep. It was hard to think he was gone.

He was tired now, and his legs ached a little as he started down the hill toward the stream. He could not see the road; it was too dark under the trees to see the sketch he had drawn. The trunks of all the trees were swollen with moss, and blowdowns blocked his way and he had to circle around their upended roots, black and misshapen. He had no idea which way Tinkhamtown was, and he was frightened. He floundered into a pile of slash, feeling the branches tear at his legs as his boots sank in, and he did not have the strength to get through it and he had to back out again, up the hill. He did not know where he was going any more.

He listened for the stream, but all he could hear was his wife, her breath catching now and then in a dry sob. She wanted him to come back, and Doc wanted him to, and there was the big house. If he left the house alone, it would fall in with the snow and cottonwoods would grow in the cellar hole. There were all the other doubts, but most of all there was the fear. He was afraid of the darkness and being alone, and not knowing the way. He had lost the way. Maybe he should turn back. It was late, but maybe, maybe he could find the way back.

And then he heard it, echoing through the air, a sound like peepers in the spring, the high silvery note of a bell. He started running toward it, following it down the hill. The pain was gone from his legs, it had never been there. He hurdled blowdowns, he leapt over fallen trunks, he put one fingertip on a pile of slash and floated over it like a bird. The sound filled his ears, louder than a thousand churchbells ringing, louder than all the heavenly choirs in the sky, as loud as the pounding of his heart. His eyes were blurred with tears, but he did not need to see. The fear was gone; he was not alone. He knew the way now. He knew where he was going.

He paused at the stream just for a moment. He heard men's voices. They were his hunting partners, Jim, Mac, Dan, Woodie. And oh, what a day it was for sure, closeness and understanding and happiness, the little intimate things, the private jokes. He wanted to tell them he was happy; if they only knew how happy he was. He opened his eyes, but he could not see the room any more. Everything else was bright with sunshine, but the room was dark.

The bell stopped, and he closed his eyes and looked across the stream. The other side was basked in gold bright sunshine, and he could see the road rising steeply through the clearing in the woods, and the apple tree in a corner of the stone wall. Cider was standing motionless, the white fan of his tail lifted a little, his neck craned forward, one foreleg cocked. The whites of his eyes showed as he looked back, waiting for him.

"Steady," he called, "steady, boy." He started across the bridge. "I'm coming."

THE SAP RAN ITS COURSE

He was a hunter, a father, a husband, a student of Buddhism, an environmentalist, a man of dignity and composure, with a capacity to communicate using words or not; a student of life, a man of command. His favorite story was *The Road to Tinkhamtown.*

He was able to maintain some control as his body became limited because his family gave this gift to him — even when he could first only whisper, and then not talk at all, and even if all he had left for most of his last days was the movement of his right arm to feed himself and his insatiable appetite from the steroids he needed to help manage the tumor expansion inside his skull.

His most demanding time was when he wanted to get up again and again in the Hoyer lift, and his family obliged, trying to relieve his energy from his sense of immobility, despite their exhaustion and incessant care. We talked about the relief of having some sense of motion in space. At that time, even getting him up became a risk for falling with more lost control of his frame. But his beloved wife was committed to giving him his freedom in the face of risking the opposite.

His processing and coming to peace with his body's decline was so full of grace, that I almost forgot the period of his loss of physical power as he realized he could no longer man his gun to protect his family. It brought fears of strangers coming into the house to get him, and images of flies coming into the windows.

Joseph's own guns were taken care of now. He invited his hunting buddy Dan over and asked him to clean them and take inventory. Dan was lean with tan hair rustled, hands callused. He had some glasses hanging on his chest that were in two parts, almost looking as if they had broken, but they were magnetized. *"Now when a beam hits them, see—"* he snapped them together and then broke the magnet connection with a thrust. He was a contractor when he was not hunting.

They talked of nature stories, laughed… like only hunting partners of thirty-plus years do. When they talked about lassoing the deer, I envisioned cowboys out West and the cattle. They laughed, *"You are not a hunter, I take it? No, we put the rope around him after he is down…"* He told of a man who lassoed a 100-pound doe that had gotten caught in his fencing, and tied the rope around himself to hold her down, thinking she was small and he'd catch her and fatten her up for venison. But the doe had more power than he anticipated, and dragged him out past the fencing until he got lucky to cut the rope and set her, and himself, free.

"They are a renewable resource," Dan said, *"Unlike the windmills they are putting up. Those are non-renewable. They only last twenty-plus years, the clearings ruin water sources for animals, the noise is bad, the roads cut through the landscape… The people who are against clear-cutting are sometimes for the windmills, but clear-cutting is renewable."* Dan and the animals are used to quiet hunting grounds.

When Dan left, Joseph got into his adjustable bed and we checked the urinary catheter, his vital signs, because his wife asked for them, absence of skin breakdown with the diligent care he received from his loved ones. Pain was well managed with him — rare headaches that were resolved often just with Tylenol.

January 9th was the first time I went to the swamp-colored green house at the end of the long dirt driveway with the sugaring shack to the side. At that time there was no wood ramp built up to its entryway. The buildings were new. The day was cold, crisp, clean. The house was warm, well-loved. A slate wood stove welcomed me. That evening Joseph talked of fighting cancer and getting better. There were already signs that the treatment was not working, but there was some question still of new avenues, and he was holding onto threads. He had made a deal with his oncologist (and friend) that if the oncologist cured him, he would give in return, the secret of growing back the hair on his bald head. Joseph was strong, confident, humorous, clear. He said later, when I asked him if he would like to record an oral history of his interesting and thoughtful life, he said no, that each person has to find that for themselves.

It was on a few visits later, when Joseph was admitted to hospice, that he said he wanted to see the syrup season through. He knew then that no new treatments were going to save him.

He was powerful, soft, rooted. To his last day, he held his role of head of the household. His wife said he was holding a lot in. I lent them a book of my friend's called Gazing at the Beloved, by Rumi. *"Interesting that you should bring that up,"* Karen said, *"Just last night I said to Joseph, 'You are talking to me with your eyes'."* He talked less and less over time, but his eyes spoke.

"I am the lucky one," he said one day before those days, looking out the window with his right eye, at the birds coming to the feeder.

What made him the lucky one? I asked, noting how he might be saying the opposite with his life ending at age fifty-seven, his terminal diagnosis of glioblastoma, and his loss of capacity to do all the physical things in life he loved — except eating (he was taking medicine that gave him a ravid appetite) and whispering to his wife and family.

"I am going to cease to exist but my family is going to continue with their burdens. And I won't be there to help them."

"What did you mean last night when you told me that you would be with me when I go to our place by the river? Were you just trying to comfort me?" Karen genuinely asked. He spoke of cellular energy, of continuity, of connection, of release, and corrected himself to say to Karen that yes, he would be with her.

The perfection of care strategies, the baking for his appetite, the interventions for the complications, the visitors, the late night talks between man and wife that became whispers without the strength to talk…

The days were surprisingly short, Karen said, and busy in that house during the months while the wife took off work to take care of her lover.

March 30th, 2013, maple sugaring season was over. March 29th, the family arranged for a maple sugaring party at the house with Joseph. The home was full of noise and laughter and busyness.

At the end of the day, the taps were pulled before everyone left.

Then it was Joseph's turn. The syrup had run. His step-mom, who had tirelessly gotten him up and down in the Hoyer lift when he felt the need to move, over and over again in every day, had gone home to rest for the night.

With his last three breaths, and with Karen lying next to his side in the small adjustable bed that she thought she could not fit in, he opened his eyes and gazed at his beloved.

The room was not dark,

and there were no flies,

as he found his way to Tinkhamtown.

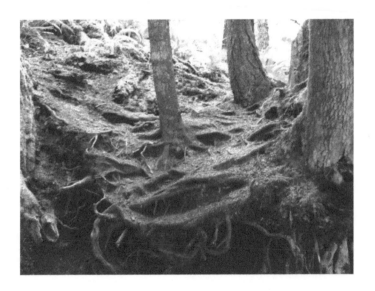

THE SHOWER

"Hi, I'm Janine." *"Hi, I'm dying."*

He was whispering because he was so short of breath and weak, That whispering was all he could do. I had never met him before. Had I misheard him? Did he have a dry sense of humor? Was he reaching out to be direct and open right from the start?

No, I had not misheard him. His wife Kaitlyn said that they were *"not like most Americans."* They have known and contemplated for a long time that they will both die. Maybe sooner than anticipated.

She was well-read on all kinds of end-of-life information, from the mundane to the inspired. She spoke of humorous writers on the physiology of death, plus serious writings from divers angles.

In 1985, when he was 43-years old, Anthony had given one of his kidneys to a dancing colleague that was a life-and-death gift for the ailing woman. He was a ballroom dancer. In 2001 his remaining kidney failed at the age of fifty nine. As a kidney donor, *"he went to the top of the list nationally"* and had a transplant after minimal dialysis. *"It lasted him seven years almost to the day,"* his wife said. *"I talk too much,"* she added. I thought she was giving me important information.

When I asked him if he had wishes, she answered for him. Then with the interruption, he couldn't remember what he was going to say... Still, it was clear that he was a man who had simple wishes: Independence and Connection.

He said he wanted to take a shower. He was barely able to get out of bed. Knowing time is not to be taken for granted, I had driven a long way to the central office to pick up a shower chair in case it could be used.

The next day when I did the Nursing Aide Intro, it felt intrusive to help with a shower just as the aide walked in and had barely met him, but we decided to go forward to maximize the possible within the impossible in limited time. Anthony wanted to take a shower, and to do it as independently as possible. That was one of his last wishes he requested in his simple, clear language.

From his improvement with the introduction of morphine in the first visit, he was now able to stand up (and breathe at the same time!). He took hold of two ski poles, and walked to the shower. The aide and I just 'spotted' him. I couldn't believe he was doing it without our hands-on help. The aide gave him a shower while I charted, and we both helped him back into his bed. The adjustable bed had arrived at the same time, from the local DME (durable medical equipment) store. (Prompt, responding within hours to requests for hospice patients). The wife did not want Anthony to use it yet.

"He has been in too many hospital beds. He hates them." I got it. *"Coming back to this bed from the hospital was one of the things he was most looking forward to. He wants to die in his own bed."*

His wife was firm. I was afraid that when/if they really needed it and decided they had to have it, that he would not be able to get up to move, and it would be too difficult to care for him. Which is what happened. But also, he got to be in his bed that first night, as he wished.

On the third day's visit, the same aide and I were at his house again. He was no longer speaking or giving eye contact. After his shower the day before, he had asked to make a number of phone calls to people with whom he said he wanted to talk. Then he became quiet.

The night before, he had hung his legs over the side and could not get them back up, nor allow her to do so — he cried out in pain when she touched him, and more so as the night went by with decreased blood flow to his dependent lower extremities. The aide has been on the ambulance crew for over thirty years. She talked to some locals. She arranged for them to come and move him to his adjustable bed with a blow-up stretcher that made his hypersensitive skin tolerate the move with minimal distress.

The adjustable bed would keep him safer and more comfortable now, and help him to be able to raise his head to administer the oral morphine, and enable aides to clean him and move him, with the air pressure mattress to relieve the pressure-points on his skin that would otherwise not get irculation.

After pre-medicating Anthony for pain, the Lift Assist crew came in with their customary mix of efficiency, skill, professionalism, comradery, sense of humor, and seriousness all at once. Kaitlyn had to step outside thinking that Anthony might cry out in discomfort. She had had all she could take of that. After we told Kaitlyn that he didn't make a sound during the process, she said, *"I should have known. They are professionals. They know what they are doing."* That was true at every level. We thanked them for making our work possible, and they were gone.

"When he first got sick, he wanted to take care of himself, Kaitlyn reminisced. *I traveled, saw my friends, lived my life instead of staying home and taking care of him. I went out and did my thing and had a good time. He gave that to me... Maybe I gave him his independence. I thought I was being a bad wife all these years, but maybe I gave him what he needed."* I agreed. He had maintained his dignity and autonomy throughout, as was still his wish when I met him.

Days later, after his death the next night, I went back to check up on Kaitlyn. I am regretfully resistant to grief visits while trying to see the living patients. I went to pick up the shower chair and bedside commode I had taken from the DME loaning shed. It was the task, I hate to admit, that got me back there. But it was Kaitlyn that gave it meaning.

"We had control," she said. *"Everyone should be able to have that as much as possible. In the hospital I lose my appetite. At home with the hospice nurses like you and David, I feel comfortable. When David came [the night before Anthony died] we talked about mountain climbing and golfing and all kinds of things. He helped ease a hard time."*

Anthony had died very comfortably with the Scopolamine patch behind the ear that helped with the tracheal congestion that came with the loss of swallowing capacity as the body function declined.

She walked out to meet me into the rainy day for the only fifteen-minute break of rain that morning. The azaleas stood out against the dark branches from the wetness.

"You gave me the time when I needed it. Now I can help you," she said. She had everything together and ready to be picked up for increased efficiency. *"I needed to do something when he was dying. By giving him the medicine, I felt like I was part of the process...*

"The only sad thing is that U.V.M. could not take his body; They have their quota. He wanted to donate his body, as you know."

We both agreed that the silver lining was in Vermonters recognizing the need for the body research, and Vermont had provided the university with that. She also said that the faster process of cremation had made it possible for their children to be part of the spreading of the ashes. *"And he didn't have to be filled up with more medicines from more needles. He has had his share of that."*

She pointed to Anthony's urn. *"I talk to him all the time. He is in there. He got the good days while he was dying,"* she said as we noted that the pouring rain had stopped. This allowed us to cram the equipment into a car that already looked filled.

"It was sunny all those last days. Now it rains... The flowers are for me,"

We noted their full bloom and iridescent brilliance.

> *"Now go to your day and spread your good will."*

"Right back to you," I said waving, back to turning on my windshield wipers.

THE SUNSET

My confidence was gone in anticipation of meeting with my supervisor to be reminded that the agency can't function financially if we don't meet the productivity numbers of more visits in less time. And I can't.

I can handle a good caseload, I can take good care of that population; I can keep up on the seemingly endless charting that is about four-fifths of the job... maybe three-fifths... and love all of it and be happy in my job, even keep healthy by taking care of myself, I think. But I cannot do it in the time the agency wants. We have lost three full-time nurses this month, we have four travel nurses... Are we ever free of travel nurse expenses? Is this working for anyone?

The sun was shining. One of those perfect spring days. I noted that I was hardly taking it in. My GPS easily took me to the next visit. The patient and his wife were on the porch taking in some sun. They had an old home that they had renovated after Hurricane Irene. The new wood floors gave a feeling of groundedness and energy at the same time.

When we went indoors because the sun was wearying the patient, who had gotten out of the hospital only a few days ago, his head hung low. Advanced renal disease. He didn't want to spend his days in dialysis, so that was dropped. A torn aorta took him to the ER. Multiple heart attacks, congestive heart-failure... His whole body ached with advanced arthritis.

His wife sat quietly across the room, giving me the chair next to him. He said he was wobbly and at times nauseous and sick of all his pills. We talked about catching the nausea before it hit. We talked about topical creams for arthritis, since he can't take anti-inflammatory medicine that upsets his stomach. We talked about improved bowel medications. He said he was taking too many pills, and that maybe they were causing the nausea. We went over the medication list. It was all pretty basic. His serious cardiac problems were the cause of much of the undeniable challenges.

I was quickly getting that the anti-depressant was not something he should be cutting out. He had two new pills, and he didn't like that. Indur, Hydralazine… they were probably making a difference in his cardio-pulmonary status, and his nausea was not new. He said he was anxious.

"You have been through a lot. You have just gotten out of the hospital. You haven't recuperated. You can't do the things you want to do. You are tired of your long history of health problems. You are sick of taking pills that you don't even know if they help, maybe they make you nauseous. You are trying to settle back in. It's a lot."

"I had a heart attack one year ago… and another one three years ago. It's going to happen again, I know that. I have had a good life, don't get me wrong. My wife is my life. She is what I live for. But if it wasn't for her, I wouldn't be here. I don't want to leave her alone. It is going to be hard for her when that time comes. She takes care of me. It's a huge burden. But she does it because she is a good woman. She is very strong. She is perfect. There is nothing else. Just her. I am only alive because of her."

He said it not with joy but with his head sunk into his chest and his eyes closed. "You are telling me that if it wasn't for her, you would not want to be alive."

"No, I wouldn't."

"Is there anything you look forward to in the morning in addition to seeing her, anything at all?"

"No. When I wake up the first thing is her. I put my arm around her. At bedtime she is my last thought."

"In addition to being with your beautiful wife, given that your life is short — we don't know how short or how long — but for a short time, is there anything you can think of that you might want to do before you die, anything you want to finish, anything that would give you a sense of purpose for your day?"

"No."

"Even if I gave you the assignment to think about it, nothing would come to mind."

"No."

"You look very discouraged."

"You would be too if you were in my shoes."

"You are right about that actually. I would be."

"I have no idea how long I am going to live — and I'm glad I don't know, I wouldn't want to know, but one time I am not going to come out of it."

"Are you scared about when that time does come?"

"No," he said as simply, clearly and assuredly as all his other 'no's'.

"Okay. I have an idea. May I invite your wife to ask you for something for herself? The reason I am asking you this is that, yes, it is a burden to take care of someone else, but also it is a great joy. It feels really good when you can do something for someone else. At the end of my day if I feel I have helped anyone, then the world feels like a better place to live in. I am sure she is tired, I am sure she gets discouraged, even when she doesn't let on. But I am also sure that it gives her great joy to give to you, because she loves you so much. So maybe there is something she would like from you, that you can give her, that would help you focus your days and give you something to look forward to."

Daniel was listening. *"He has a grandson,"* Regina said.

"What do you like to do with your grandson?" I asked Daniel.

"I like to spend time with him. I like to make him laugh."

"Okay. There's one thing. What about for you?" I asked Regina.

"Like what kind of thing?" Regina asked me.

"Anything," I said. "Wives often have something they would really like from their husbands that they stop asking for because it becomes too much trouble. Something he can still do."

"He knows that I really like sunsets. I like to go to the waterfront and watch the sunset."

"Are you able to get in a car?" I asked Daniel. I had just met him and didn't know him very well.

"Yes. She drives."

"Is that something you could do?"

"Yes. I think I see where you are going."

"Ok. This is your assignment: I will help you keep your body going as long as it can. That is my job as your nurse. You work every day to keep yourself as strong and well as you can, so that at the end of the day you might be able to get in the car with your wife and go see a sunset with her. And your job is to spend as much time as you can with your grandson."

"I think you are onto something."

"It is going to be hard. It is much easier to sink into the misery of your situation. You have a lot of misery to think about. But now you have a gift you can give your wife. And your grandson. Now your life can be rich. You are going to be engaged because you have a purpose. The hard part is not going to go away, but your life is going to be good, even with all your health problems. If it is one day, two days, if it is two weeks, or two years, it will be hard, and it will also be good."

They were both crying.

"You have helped us,"

Daniel said as I gathered my bags from their beautiful wood floors. I walked into the sunshine to get him a condom catheter from the back of my car, so he might sleep through the night.

He got up and was walking with the support of his walker.

I got into my mobile automobile office, as I call it, reaching for my seat belt… Daniel had gotten up and had not forgotten his walker, his head was far from his chest. He was smiling.

I drove to my next visit through the beautiful Mad River Valley. Now I felt present in the day. The dreaded weekly probation meeting with my boss had gotten lost in giving myself to someone else's pain.

That night Daniel died.

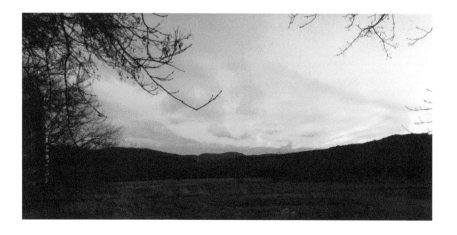

LIVING

It was at a Spanish hardwood table that Sharon and Glendon sat
when I came back home from my trip to Spain.
Their 45th wedding anniversary was coming up June 29th, they said.

As I called for new medication orders and the doctor's line was on hold,
I asked them how they had met.
Her sister had introduced them they said. "How?" I asked.
Sharon said that her sister worked with him
and brought him over to the house.

"I told my sister that night
that he was the last man on earth that I would go out with."

Glendon felt the same:
"I said I wouldn't take her to the back house if she was the only woman around."

"So what happened?" I asked.
Clearly I wasn't going to get much out of them without pressing.

"We met six months later and it was different."

"How did you meet six months later?"
Getting a story out of a Vermonter
felt like the drips of maple syrup from their trees.

*"What happened is that we were in a car after a dance.
You and I were in the back,"* she said, looking at her husband, *"*
*Then he nailed me across the back seat and smacked a kiss on me.
And we went from there."*

"It was coming into East Montpelier just before that 'yield' sign that's there,"
he said.

"Now it is said we are in the golden years. I am not sure what that means,"
Sharon commented.

"The golden years have come at last.
I get it why they call it that —
They're taking all the gold I have
To pay for all I cannot do:
I cannot see, I cannot pee
I cannot chew, I cannot screw
Oh my God, what can I do??
My hearing stinks, my memory shrinks
No sense of smell, I look like hell.
My body's drooping,
Got trouble pooping.
My mood is bad, as can you tell ~
The golden years have come at last!
The golden years can kiss my ass."

Her husband could barely breathe behind the oxygen tube in his nose.
He suffered acute cardiac exacerbations daily, his muscle-mass was wasted.
His hemorrhoid bleeding had gone through six pads
post an episode of constipation that was secondary
to the morphine before he started on the miralax…
and before the blood thinner was stopped.

Still, his eyes laughed, as did hers when she looked at him, and he teased.
He said he wanted to live, not die. He did not want to talk about dying.
They looked across the table that they bought at an auction
in their first year of their marriage, saying they don't need new furniture
when what they have is still strong.
"A lot stronger than the wood composites they make today."

"New shit? Kiss my ass," his wife said. Glendon winked at her.

DYING

A few days later, Glendon's wife said he wasn't well.

I found him in a back room crying tears that were honestly soaking the floor
as he sat forward with his elbows on his knees.

I could barely understand the words that were drowned into his chest.

In broken parts and syllables, he said he wanted to be there for his wife and
family, and that when he dies he won't be able to.

He said he wasn't ready to die but that he thought he was dying anyway.

We talked about death on that visit,
and what he imagined after-death would be like.

He said it would be nothing.

His wife walked into the room.

We talked about families who say they remain connected
to their loved ones after they die.

He said he knew that they would have memories.

I told him about my dad, who thought there would be nothing after death,
despite being Catholic, and how every one of his children had found profound
ways in which he is still in our lives, and that he is still helping us.

His wife said that they knew where he was going.
They had strong religious convictions.

On the next visit Sharon said that Glendon had lead his family in hymns
after he had a dream of gold
"That was more beautiful than could be imagined," he said.
The house was still packed with people when I got there.
He told his grandchildren about his dream and said that
there was no need to be afraid of death.

He said he had no trouble breathing, no bleeding, no chest pains.

His medications and treatment interventions were in balance.
He was sitting at his place at the Spanish oak dining table
where we usually met. He was relaxed and teasing.
His face wrinkles smiled.

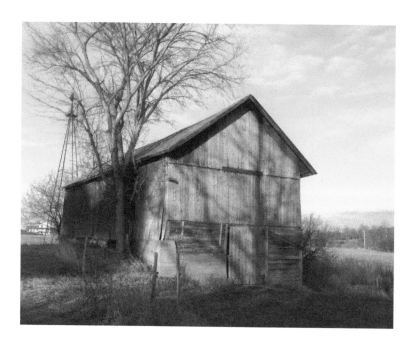

GOING HOME

I didn't tell you that at 8-years-old Glendon got stuck in a silo
and almost lost his breath.
When he was a bit older, he had a bout of kidney failure, they said.
His last months now, brought that back.

He talked to his wife about the farm.
In his sleep he milked the cows with hand movements.
"We haven't had cows for years," his wife said.
He continued to have dreams.

"Sparkling wings and bright colors of pinks,
purples, red with pinkish-colored stripes of gold…
Ain't anything here like it, and it's much prettier than I'm telling you."

Between them was his fears of leaving his family with unmet care needs.
On long days he would say,

"Every day is the same… Just waiting for the day to come…
Then I'm going to jump hula-hoops."

At one point, his dreams got disturbing enough to need the help of Haldol
—a medication that soothes fears and bad dreams
and helps people relax into the natural process
of saying good-bye to this world.
(In hospice it does not have time for the untoward longer-term side effects.)

Next he was telling his family and friends of the gold
that made death something, *"No one should be afraid of."*

One day he said he'd take a bar of soap and go out in the downpour
during the spring of excessive rain. He teased even when his breath was short.

"They're weird dreams: Last night I went to a church and I couldn't find her;
she couldn't find me; I could see all these people... no one could tell me where she
was; we couldn't get back together... "

Sharon said, *"He said he wanted to go home."* Glendon added, *"I don't know*
which home I want to go to. I know I am going to the Lord's home...
I don't want to go yet."

I told him that if he was not ready yet, then he was probably not going yet.
That was three weeks before he died. At the next visit he said,
"I got a call at 2am from someone looking for a dentist.
I told them to take two aspirin and call me back in the morning.
They didn't call back.
If they had, I would have told them to get some pliers and get rid of the thing.
—That's what I tell my grandchildren when they come around
saying they have a toothache from eating too much candy."

His wife tended to every need. He wanted to die in his own bed, not an
adjustable bed. That makes lifting the head hard, and moving the body hard,
for cleaning and for improved breathing and for giving medicines.
It makes getting out of bed to the bedside commode hard,
skin breakdown issues hard.

She managed it all.

Except for her tired red eyes, she never let on to being stressed and grieving,
until after we started the morphine pump when she hadn't slept all night.
He had broken a fever overnight in profuse sweat.
When he was quiet with the pump effective, then she and her daughter
were submerged in their exhaustion and long days of patience,
and work, and sleeplessness.

"We held a circle of arm holds and allowed the silence to do its own work."
"A man in white is going to come and get me," Gordon proclaimed one day.

My guess is that is how it went. He said so.

SO MANY

Many others I have not told you about.

About the man whose history was of decades of sexual abuse to his children, one of whom was a close friend of mine: How she came in the day he died, and for the first time she could see that he no longer had power over her.

About the homeless woman who didn't know how to take comfort or know how to receive.

About Chester Pierce who called his girl "Curlicue" and whom our one male nurse colleague called a 'pisser'. I can't believe I have not written Chester's story. The reason is that he lives his life so beyond my page that you would have to go to his living room and listen to his story, in his own loud, crisp, indisputable conviction and energy.

I think I missed my cue in making him the story teller. You wouldn't have been able to put his book down. I would have had to sit with my computer or with a tape recorder to capture his style. Even then it wouldn't have the same impact as his presence. When alluding to his hope of healing: *"I shall be able to leap from tall buildings in a single bound."*

Or the time a new doctor looked at his chart full of notes about his nephrostomy tubes, his ostomy bag, his urinary catheter (that was hidden unusually neatly under his pant leg), his abdominal drain in a large abdominal incision epithelializing, the hole in his bladder that made him pee out his rectum… "You don't look like the man I am reading about," the doctor spoke frankly.

"Oh yea?" he said, throwing up his shirt and revealing his wounds and tubes, *"Appearances can be deceiving."* What was not deceiving was Chester's charm and humor was his on-target self advocacy and determination to get back to his craft of making knives, and get back to living without tubes.

I didn't tell you about the sudden death of a high school friend David: Bright, in great physical shape, a leading lawyer looked up to by many and loved for his wit and cleverness and warmth… Who died suddenly on the treadmill from a heart attack, after being told he had a clean bill of cardiac health, now leaving behind his beloved wife and children. Along with the heart-wrench, he left his huge laughter and generosity of spirit that he wore in his cowboy boots.

I haven't told you about the beautiful woman on the cover of this book who was a patient of ours and was related to David — that high school friend who was also my first boyfriend, and who was going to come over to dinner last night for a high school reunion with his wife and my beloved high school friend Mary who flew home from Jakarta where she works for public health. Mary and I walked to the rushing brook on the other side of the covered bridge yesterday, and talked as we did over thirty-five years ago in the same high school where I met David. A lifetime of hours were between, and none at all. (Mary took the photo of me on the back sleeve of the book.)

Betsy Eckfeldt, the woman on the cover, wanted to visit her son one last time. She knew the rest of the visits would be him visiting her. On the way back, she needed to rest before reaching her bed. She sat on that porch of hers, where I asked her if I could take her picture. When I admired the photo, I asked her if I could use it on the cover of my book. She was excited about that.

Then Susan Steele's words, the sister-in-law of a patient: *"You just need people to hear, you don't need a lot of other stuff."*

And another family member, as I acknowledged the family care-giving demands: *"If she can go through this, we can."*

My hairdresser said, *"The people you think will be there for you are not the ones that necessarily come through. And sometimes it's strangers that are there for you."*

I haven't told you about the woman who was hidden inside of huge folds of flesh that, despite my being physically strong, I didn't have the strength to lift and clean under when she got yeast infections in the folds, and how inside, beyond that, there was someone who was free of all that weight, but who was hidden in her shell. About her small husband who took care of her day in and day out, and how he drank in between. They took over their own care, by request, so I stopped seeing them. The many birds in the tight room were the ones she felt understood by, I think. How they managed when they discovered that her husband was allergic to the birds, I don't know. Their life was hard. She seemed absent. But again, she was under there somewhere, and could be seen in seconds when a glint in her eye shone. She taught me that.

I didn't tell you about Fernanda Mason who is in her 90's who has dementia and whose body holds on one day to the next and who doesn't understand the possibility — to say nothing of the concept — of complaint.

She sits in her chair watching the horses out her window, with flies buzzing around her and her food crumbs fallen over her lap and floor as she feeds her meals to her dog.

"I am disgustingly healthy." Or on the next visit she says, *"I am disgustingly happy. I can sit here all day and watch the horses... You take the good with the bad... Now the horse is going back to the barn."* The animals in her life are as important to her as her niece who had taken her in. One Vermont day after another passes by her window, and she sits there taking it in, not finding anything negative to think, it seems.

We keep wondering if she is going to need hospice services instead of the current Palliative Care services, but every time she gets a bad cold or dizzy spells or a urinary tract infection, and looks like she's not going to make it, she comes back to her old self – well, almost.

I didn't tell you about getting called into room 113 to pronounce a woman dead, and fumbling for a light when I got there. *"May I help you?"* the dead woman in the bed said. The room I was supposed to have gone into was not 113. It was 116. The nurse who directed me to the wrong room, with a live person it, thought that was funny. I laughed too… but not when I startled at the voice.

I didn't tell you about my colleague who could not make her deceased mother's Beef Stroganoff to taste like her mom's, so she asked Dolly, who was a good cook.

This patient often used our first name throughout her sentences, showing her respect and warmth. Dolly gave her the tips and also the special bouillon for the broth. My friend called the cook in tears that night, gratefully thanking her for the giving of Mother's Stroganoff. Two weeks later the wonderful woman died (not my colleague), having had another moment of being her own person and being needed, useful, wanted. And my friend has the memory of this beautiful person coupled with Mother's love.

Finally, on a night I needed a chuckle, Perkins Funeral Home in Vermont told me that they are the last ones to let us down and that we get a walk-in discount when it is our turn. Imagine that.

"Life goes on," said the widow Karen Organto,
"It is always startling."

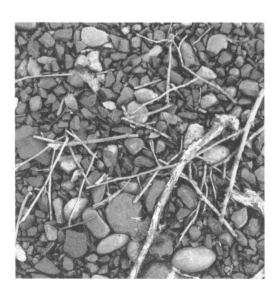

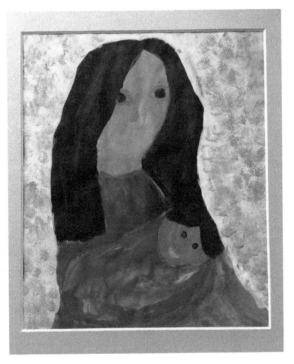

© Art by Samantha Carranza

MOTHERS

I borrow mothers as I go
accepting love for far away sons and
distant daughters
as my own.
I hold other mothers' hands and look
them in the eyes and in these moments
we belong.
They let me tuck them into bed
and kiss their cool dry cheeks and
in return I hold still
to let them
push a stubborn strand of hair out of my eyes.
I let the stolen tenderness sweep over me, and
hope that far away
another son or daughter is
using my mother
as their own.

~ Mary Brutsaert, LCSW

I'VE AWOKEN

I've awoken
in this bed of poppies,
bereft,
to a water colored,
paper thin dawn.

Tanagers, and sweet
warblers burst
brightly between
the warm, whispered
low, soft coos of
collared doves.

Half of me awake, soothed
beneath this downy comforter,
the other half asleep
and expanding indefinitely
beyond the freshly lit horizon.

Good morning,
good bye,
and this chorus
all sound
exactly the same.

~ R Daley Jr MA

Part Five

THE VALLEY
OF CONTENTMENT

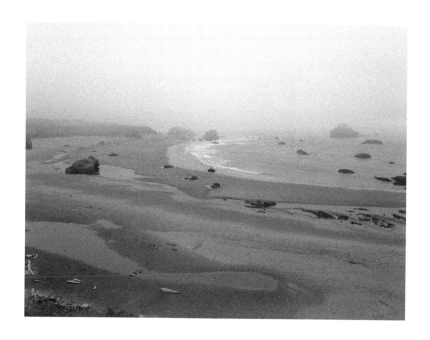

At Peace

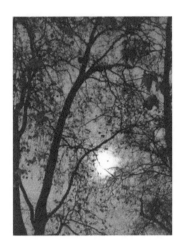

When the dead are honoured
and when the memory of the most distant ancestor remains alive,
the strength of a people attains its fullest expression.

~ Confucius

SEEING THE STARS

The elderly woman reached over the banister of the raised porch on the assisted living facility as the sun shone over her. She was picking off the dead flowers growing in pots. Well, some of the ones not-dead too, to be honest — either from poor eyesight, poor dexterity, or from excessive delight in the fresh ones, I don't know.

Leaving from a visit, I walked through the wood gate with a hook-and-eye latch, and a large notice to '*please remember to latch the door*'. Just on the other side of the gate were some large white and lavender-tinged flowers multitudinously in bloom, covering the vine. I gave myself permission, not only to pick one of the flowers, but to also to go back and give it to this elderly woman who lived in the same place as the new patient I had just visited. We chatted pleasantly for a minute, sharing the beautiful day and the priority to notice it and make it a happy one.

On my next visit, I wheeled Linda, a 102-year-old patient, out to watch the moon rise, wrapped in a fleece blanket, while I assessed her condition and wrote my nursing note. The doorman brought her hot tea in an unsolicited gesture of presence and caring. It was the night of the harvest moon. Linda sang,

> "*There's a moon, way up high; here are you and here am I.*"

> "*I haven't seen the stars in ages,*" she said.

She used to ski every week and can't get enough of the out of doors — now or before.

> "*I wonder if I could still ski,*" she said.

Yes, 102-years-old. We promised to meet again, the door man and us, at the harvest moon next year. The woman gracefully said,

"That would be lovely."

In the end, both she and I had moved on by the next anniversary of that moon. But I went back to see her the next night and took her outdoors for our visit to see the sunset. Despite having seen the stars with her on the previous night, she said again,

"It has been years since I have seen the stars."

It was the same with the sunset: After fifteen minutes of being back inside, she had forgotten the outing. She hadn't forgotten me or the watchman, though. Nor her sons who visited her frequently.

I kissed her goodnight and went back out the latched gate, closing it carefully.

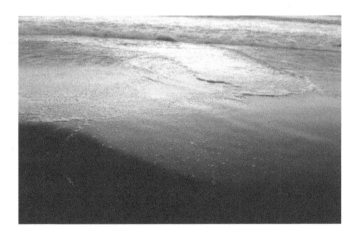

HOLDING HANDS IN THE DARK

When the outside world is roiling

Like a splashing, crashing sea

And inside the anger's boiling

Crying "Set me free!"

When your loves go to a stranger,

Staccato shot through a working day,

Coming home you dance with danger

And loved ones - you've nothing to say.

Heartfelt connection is what you crave

While tired is what you feel.

It's me, you think, I need to save

And feed on something real.

The crashing sea it ebbs and flows

And tides they rise once more.

Unexpected kindness comes, and shows

A sunny peaceful shore.

~ Troy Maddux, LMT

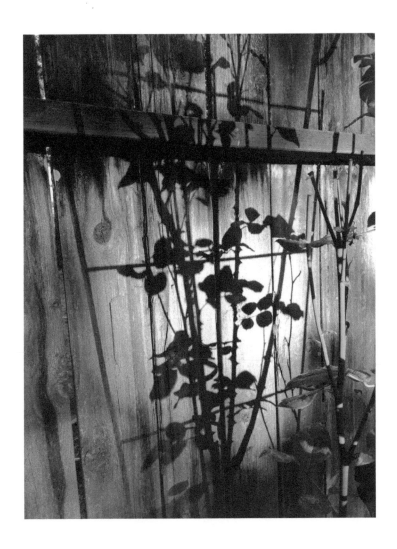

SO FAR I REALLY LIKE DYING

Sogie is the helper monkey, not the patient. She pats the side of her wire room hard when I come in, alerting me that she knows I am an intruder to her small circle of friends.

There is a film-clip of Sogie and Jade, done by a National Geographic photographer, with Sogie helping Jade pick up dropped things and putting them back in her pocket, and turning on and off light switches for Jade. The monkey sees Jade as herself, and as a companion — not as a disabled body.

Getting Sogie to come into the home legally with the State of Vermont was a difficult battle. Sogie was still considered a wild animal, despite being trained as a helper monkey, and as such against the law in a residence. But Jade and her husband Gordon got their way in the end, and were allowed to welcome the trained monkey helper. Gordon wouldn't take no for an answer.

He is a contractor and indomitable man, with one of his love-languages being the persistence of getting Jade what she has needed for twenty-eight years after she was diagnosed with multiple sclerosis months following their marriage. Sogie became family.

"It's been good with us," Gordon said about his family. I told him it was obvious. *"But I feel robbed out of twenty years with her. I am monstrously bitter about that,"* he said with gritty emphasis. He spoke of the dread of the day he would lose her and lose Sogie too when Sogie's official job was done.

They met on a boat and within two days, were talking about marriage. She said she knew he was the man the moment she saw him. A few things got in the way in the next years before they did get married, but nothing bigger than what they have faced all their years together. This weekend is their 28th wedding anniversary.

Every last detail and process of care for Jade is finessed toward the result of Jade lying in her bed or sitting up in her chair looking like she can move when in fact the last movement she has remaining below her neck is a slight movement of her right hand. The blue tube that circles to her face, connected to a bag made for IV's, enables Jade to drink water as desired, when desired. Gordon and Jade figured that out together. Like so many other things two bright minds can figure.

The adjustable bed that arrived was for a single person, not a married couple in love. The durable medical equipment suppliers still don't provide the double adjustable beds for the hospice benefit. Gordon didn't like it, and he said so. It looked like an intruder to the queen-sized bed with the memory-foam mattress that had warmed them for short and long nights. By the next visit an adjacent, neatly-fitting extension to the adjustable bed transformed the intrusion. Gordon didn't waste time, as he didn't have time on his side.

A few months earlier, Gordon transcribed these words for Jade as she spoke:

So far I really like dying.
I hope it doesn't get nasty.
My people are bright constellations.
They're stars.
I'm so full — I'm really full,
Imagine.
I think I'm winding up life on an excellent note.
It's been a gas.
Willie said it was the people in this life.
He always said that —
He never finished the sentence.
I get it now.

Today Jade said that she feels like she is reducing. Then said that while her body reduced she also felt like she was expanding. She said letting the body go is like the transition in birth where in birthing, one is sure to not be able to do it — that it will kill them.

She talked about how hard it is to no longer be able to read and do the things that she used to do in alone-time. Her voice is her sparse remaining control beyond her active and subtle mind. Now even her words sometimes slip. Her smile doesn't. And Sogie doesn't.

It may be time to be calling Islene Runningdeer, the 'other-world' music therapist, to help Jade with her death song.

Gordon said it is inconceivable to imagine life after Jade and Sogie are gone. Truly inconceivable. He runs two bodies day and night, since Jade's is immobile and his is not. It is when I see her skin that I get the tiniest window into what he does. Her skin is like peaches, for want of a better cliché. Soft, pink, with no breakdown even with the low body mass and bony protrusions. Usually when a family shows me skin problems, it is a pressure sore, a skin tear. With her, they show me a little bug bite, a tiny blood vessel that broke. She remains a beauty queen in all aspects.

Gordon said today that he talked to a man who has re-built his life after the inconceivable of his wife dying. *"He says it is completely different. It is nothing like what it was before."*

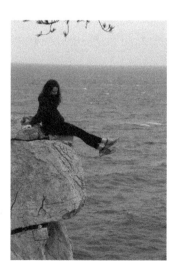

CRASHING

The helper monkey was sucking on her fist in the corner of the room. *"She is self-comforting. She is giving us our private time,"* Jade whispered. Jade was lying flat in bed. I was leaning over the bed from a stool with my elbows on her mattress. Our talk was soft, direct, open. We were listening to the universe, listening to each other, navigating daily functioning for its maximum capacity.

As we closed our visit, Jade said, *"I think we have a good plan now. If it changes and turns out to be a dumb plan, we'll exchange it for an equally brilliant plan."* I felt like Jade and Gordon understood hospice better than I did.

My next visit was in response to Gordon's call that Jade had decided to not eat and drink, that they had hit a wall together. Jade had just had a small bowl of oatmeal. Yesterday food was an aversion; she was certain she would never eat and drink again in order to speed up this dying process. Then why was she craving oatmeal this morning?

"I don't want to be crying wolf," she said in distress, confusion, conflicting emotions, tears, swirling thoughts and unclear direction in the face of the unknown timing of her death. I told her that there is only one measure I know of to direct when-what-how-much to eat and drink in the dying process, and that is: What she wants. (Short of VSED — 'Voluntarily Stopping Eating and Drinking,' to force your body to die sooner.)

The path is neither predictable nor pre-determinable by any one or anything I know, nor easy nor straightforward, nor right nor wrong. Professional measures are not in control. Her wishes rule. I reminded her that in the end, dying dry is the most comfortable death, just as living with liquid is the most comfortable in life. Because at the end the body loses its capacity to manage liquid and takes it to the wrong places, like the heart and lungs and into puffing-up the extremities and other places, with unwanted fluid. The delineation between comfort in liquid or comfort in dryness is marked by loss of appetite and loss of thirst. Our bodies know this transition and give us the message.

When she asked how to know the timing of when she is going to die, the best that can be offered to meet the unique individuality of mind, body, and spirit is that when a body is changing in significant ways monthly, that one has roughly months to live; when weekly, roughly weeks to live; when daily, days; when hourly, hours. For all but sudden events like a heart attack, stroke, car accident, etc. (of course), the physical body find its way to unite with the will, the spirit, the emotions, and the good-bye to this life. Then it is time to move on. The infinite diversity, complexity, nuances, and moving parts in each one of us, for body and spirit meeting up for death timing, is the reason it is true that the most experienced professional cannot call time.

There were still harder hurdles to get through on this round. Earlier in the visit while she was still sitting up in her chair, she could hardly talk through her tumultuous emotions and her already shallow breaths. Her air volume was shortchanged for breath and voice, even when she was not feeling emotional.

"I am just a taker. I suck everything out of people. I don't give out, I just take. I suck out the energy in people." Her words rolled out chunk by chunk as a carpet of agonizing entreat, into the quiet room where I sat with my knees scrunched up on a stool next to her wheelchair and Gordon sat on the floor with his back to the refrigerator, arms crossed over his chest, and his legs stretched out in front of him. Gordon and I listening and telling her what she means to us felt like a drop compared to this effulgence of emotional pain — Hopefully a little consoling.

On another visit, Jade was looking out after the various caregivers that were in her room at the same time, knowing and keeping track of each one and their needs. She had developed this skill and grace over many years. I commented, "Jade, you're keeping track of each of us, and taking care of all of us."

"Of course," she said, *"That's my job,"*

"I thought you said you are just a taker?" She started to cry.

"*Thank-you,*" she said, and cried harder. "*Did you hear what she said, Gordon?*"

"*Yes.*" Gordon said. And she cried more.

Sogie was making noise and holding out a syringe. She wanted it filled with peanut butter. With permission from Jade, I took the syringe.

"*Back off!*" Jade said urgently. "*She is upset now.*"

I had over-stepped my boundaries in the family. It was time for me to leave and allow the monkey to re-establish her territory. I asked Jade if I could call on her when she was gone.

"*Just say, 'Send me a chicken!' and then watch,*" she said. "*When you see a chicken in a totally inappropriate place, then you will know I am close by. Did you know that? Chickens are my connection here.*"

On the way out to my car, after three hours and the need to answer my pager, Gordon said, "*I am torn between wanting her to live forever and wanting her to die tomorrow.*" He shared that when Jade had awoken not-dead that morning, as she did every morning lately, and as he repositioned her per their elaborated routine, she had said to him, "*Don't breathe in my face!*"

"*That hurt my feelings really bad,*" Gordon had said as he accompanied me to my car. "*I didn't understand that at all. What is with that, anyway? Aside from the fact that I wasn't even breathing in her face?*"

"Maybe she is asking for her private time in her last days," I conjectured. "I think there is a time when we say goodbye to our lives in private without relating directly to others. Maybe she was trying to do that in that moment. Maybe she was trying to take that space."

Gordon pondered. I opened my car door. "*Oh, and by the way,*" Gordon said as it started to rain with some energy, and as he picked up the mail in his mailbox, "*That stuff about taking care of myself is bullshit. Everyone says that. I can do anything for a short time.*" Jade and many others had been asking him to do something for himself (for a long time). "*I need that from you,*" Jade had said.

On my next call to Gordon, I had been thinking more about the comment she had made about her not wanting him to breathe in her face in that moment. I told him about delivering my second child at home, and when my then 10-year-old daughter walked into the room a little before I transitioned in the birthing. I remember feeling a turmoil at her entrance. I wanted to tend to my daughter's needs and her certain uncertainty in walking in when I was vocal in the birthing process, in the most intense part of birthing. Kate, my oldest daughter, had not had the slow ascendance of the already many hours of labor while she was at school. I couldn't help her. I was having too hard a time on my own. If I had been out with my feelings, I might have said, "Don't breathe in my face," even if she wasn't breathing in my face. I couldn't tend to her needs and feelings and I felt an excruciating conflict inside me of wanting to be there for her and having to be there for me and a new baby.

"I wonder if Jade needs space to focus on dying, between all the time that she desperately needs you to care for her. I wonder if she needs space in pieces, in-between, when she can birth herself into her next phase of life, and when she knows you are okay. She's trying to take care of you too." Jade had spoken with a directness: *"I am saying it for myself: I want Gordon to do something for himself for ME. I am the only thing he has. I want him to have other things."*

"Maybe Jade cannot die until she sees you happy taking care of yourself," I said. "Maybe that is why she said that she needs that. While she needs to find her space to let go, she may need to know that you will also find yours."

Gordon was listening. After pulling away from the phone three times to answer Jade's calls, he said, *"I am hearing what you are saying. I just had a long talk with a friend psychologist who practically beat me up telling me that I have to take care of myself. It is probably not an accident that you are calling me telling me this just two hours after."*

A few times in the next days, he tried (sort of) to do things for himself when there was a caregiver in the house. But new needs arose: New night-care needs started to keep him from sleeping night after night. Before now, there was time at least for sleeping. When the base of relief in sleep was also taken, his emotional and physical world came crumbling down. He crashed. His years of strength and resolve and innovation and resilience dissolved in an instant. Gordon had physically and emotionally and spiritually collapsed.

Out of desperation, he finally asked for help. He got overnight help, and slept. The response of overwhelming love, in the genuine form of practical help and sincere expression, made a shift with him and Jade. He had also called the music therapist, Islene Runnigdeer: *"I told her we were having a hard time. She came over. She played Bach for a long time. And then she left."*

The house smelled like incense. They said it was from a ceremony they had just completed, where he and Jade had renewed their vows. There was a calm in the air that told me I was not needed. *"People should tell each other when they love you,"* Jade said. *"I didn't know there were so many who care about us."*

Gordon added, *"It has taken me 65 years to shift. I have always been someone who thinks I can do everything myself. It took crashing.*

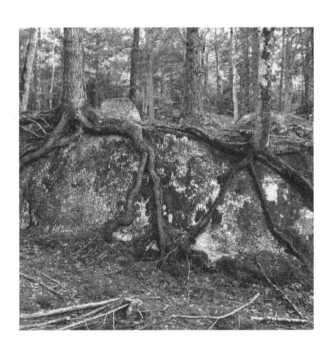

SIX SINKS
AND A CIRCUS MONKEY

"Savage wistfulness haunts me." Gordon had read these words that spoke to his state of grief. *"Indefatigable neediness"* were words that spoke to him from a book he read about caring for an ill partner.

Her ashes sat on the dining room table. He said he was trying to come to terms with that. *"She had a funny sense of humor and funny mental frame."* He spoke of adventures of daring in his 20's:

"I would turn off the lights of what I was doing and basically lock the door and walk away and go off into another world of drama and fear and excitement and high energy and the strong potential of death, and I thought nothing of it. I could sail through typhoons and shoot pirates, all in a day's work. And now at the age of 65, the idea of getting out of my own shadow is getting me a little bolloxed.

When I was sailing we'd be caught in some awful storm. Storms happen and you deal with them. You'd be scared shitless and say, 'I hope that wave doesn't fall on me… Oh my Lord! Well, I have seen worse than this. This isn't the worst storm I have ever seen. I got through it the last time so I should be ok.' And then it was some newly defined 'worst storm' and I would be terrified. I'd think, 'What am I doing out here? This is total insanity.'

In a way, that mindset — though perverse — served me in good stead with Jade. Because I didn't care. When shit happened, I said, 'I can do that.' Except with Jade, it only got worse. I didn't have the luxury of standing on my laurels from my previous experience: I couldn't count on this as a doable thing. I would say, 'I can do this,' Then it would dive into new some new unheard-of depth. 'Are you serious? Now you can't even wiggle your fingers to drive the wheelchair at all??? Does that mean you are going to be in bed the rest of life? Or me pushing your wheelchair the rest of your life??'

The loss for both of us was brutal. And it happened time and time again... You know that aluminum custom-made sink we have in the bathroom? That is the sixth sink. Each sink was perfect. It did everything we needed it to do at that particular time. That particular time was short-lived. Her feet would go too far and run into the wall and she'd get black toes — toes that were already black...

Then she'd smash her knees on the bottom of the sink. Then the next sink was perfect. She could get far enough under it so she wouldn't spit on herself, then something else would shift and I'd rip it out and do it again. Then that bizarre sink, at that stage in her process, was the perfect sink. We both took delight in that. Just before it all went to hell at the end.

If she lived for a couple of more months, it would have been # 7, or 8. All diseases must have their quirks, but MS has to be high on the quirk scale. There were more issues, and it got to be harder. I remember when Jade was diagnosed and she said, 'I can deal with squiggly handwriting, but when I can't go to the bathroom on my own any more, I'm done.' How little we knew what was ahead of us. That has been the least of it. Everything went crazy all the time. I am always trying to fix stuff, but it was constant, over and over again."

Facing conjuring up a new life after the death of his companion and partner, the *"magnetic enticer,"* as he called her, of the many deeply connected people in their life, was much harder than his dangerous trips of old, around the world, he said.

"I can fix a screen door. I can put in a new sink that works. That is my expertise. I am a contractor. My father is a mechanical engineer. Our constant refrain was, 'So what is the worst-case scenario?' and we work back from that. It's not like that now."

At the wake, Jade's boyfriend of old, and friend of always since, said:

"On our way to the Caribbean in 1981, we picked up a letter from her at one of the mail drops. It was long and newsy, handwritten on a yellow legal pad. In the middle of page 2, in parentheses, she wrote: 'Look at what just happened to my handwriting there. What's up with that?'

She hadn't met Gordon yet. That would happen a couple of months later when she joined us in St. Martin and we went to St Barth's in search of Bear Dagan. But that wobble in her handwriting was the handwriting on the wall. She was going to need someone truly extraordinary. Not just someone with a bottomless reservoir of love, but someone with an amazingly fortunate set of talents, to keep bushwhacking a path for her: Building an elevator to keep her mobile and free, a kitchen to keep her cooking, raised garden beds to keep her in basil, a bathroom to preserve her dignity, a sun-room to lift her spirits — Steadily transforming your home to stay one leap ahead of her relentless illness.

But in a powerful twist, that fateful day, when you, Gordon, first parted the banana fronds to greet us, there was so much more that needed to unfold. She first had to be that unwavering support for you. We're used to thinking about how people support each other through the day-to-day of their lives together. But I don't know of another story like yours and Jade's, where, for the entire arc of your time together you have been each other's pillar in such a magnificent swap of fortitude."

Gordon pondered in his kitchen that would no longer serve Jade: *"I don't want to just wear the new suit Jade left me, but I am afraid of the changes ahead."* Islene and I both saw Gordon's capacity for taking on new "clothing", learning to internalize and transform with it, not only in time, but usually even without delay.

"There is so much potential resistance to this kind of talk," Gordon said. *"It is like being a hopeless drunk and then for whatever reason deciding to not be a hopeless drunk anymore and you don't have anyone to talk to about anything. You've got a whole other crew who holds different values than the crew you are used to. It is ridiculously difficult. It is daunting spiritually.*

It has been heavy sledding. I don't want to do that all the time. I might break something. It's the opposite of the least common denominator; it's in the width of it — It's in the width of a life that the growth and the magic happens. If in fact the key to this is connection with other people, then you better get good at that. You'd better learn how. But I'm not good at that; I'm a wallflower. I won't have any help around that stuff without Sogie and Jade. Our friends are primarily Jade's friends. I came on the scene and it felt a lot like I was accepted because I was the husband.

I came with the package.

We gifted each other. It was a stupendous marriage. If you were looking for sad parts, it would be that it took me so long to realize how stupendous it was. There was the time in her last days when she told me I should learn to listen to others and not have to do things my way. At first I wanted to defend myself and say, 'Really?? You're going to rake me over the coals after I just changed your diaper for the fourth time? You have to do this NOW??' But then I got it. She wanted to give me advice while she still could. Before it was too late. I get it now.

It's the same old shit: Connection. Nothing else is broad-based enough to hit all the facets. The challenge is to be big-hearted . Manage to be big-hearted in the broadest sense of the word. And I don't trust any one."

It had been Zail Berry, MD, their hospice doctor, who had given them permission, before Jade died, to experience simultaneously divergent and seemingly conflicting feelings.

Gordon kept a journal for the closing three days of "her body's useful life." He wrote steadily on those days in the early hours of the mornings. He said he had not done much writing, but that it came clearly and evenly.

THURSDAY

4am morphine
Stayed up listening to J.
Eventually the sun came up directly over the barn
— Totally clear day with Camel's Hump outlined
and just as the sun appeared,
there was the momentary thought to just keep staring at it.
Throughout the day J's breathing dominated everything.
Sometimes laboring sometimes a soft breeze whispering
by her vocal cords on its way by.
It was a quiet whistling like a north wind.

All the docs indicated a fairly imminent death
with all the usual caveats
about 'we really don't know when'.
Hospice Doc stopped by;
said there was nothing medical to be done,
kissed me, kissed Jade + left.

It's now 11pm +
the breath sounds are close to those from 12 hours ago.
I waver between absolute assurance that everything is ok,
that all is well,
that everything is perfectly on time; + total panic.
How do you create a life
when suddenly 1/2 of it disappears in an instant?
I assume I'll figure it out.
Millions of other people seem to have done it.
But it doesn't seem sensible.
Like fish riding bicycles.
When J is beside me,
yet so obviously in a completely different context,
I picture her as a multi-colored reef fish
lazily swimming deep, deep in the sea.
Then the timbre of her breathing changes
and she's back beside me, more or less.
I'd like to be holding her when she really goes
but wonder whether it really matters —
In a flash she will, in her estimation,
be in another world so different,
so bright, so wonderful as to be actually incomparable.
Her faith in the hereafter
is so much more complete, intact, nuanced,
that I hope she is right
and that I can tag along on her coattails
even if heaven isn't + her end really is the end.

I am so glad that I've experienced her early finale.
We've worked so hard + so long
to have her life come to a close in our home,
in our bed with our cats, with our monkey.
This has been our plan for years + it's finally coming to pass
just as we'd hoped.
This stuff is enormously hard physically + emotionally
+ it could be argued by some that the smart $
would spring for a professional environment
run by professional folks.
But not me.
After helping J. for so many yrs,
to miss the final installment would be awful.
The whole process has been so full, so rich, so loamy,
I wouldn't trade it for anything.

Staying awake, watching her breathe,
waiting with her to her final breath,
is my last gift to her.

FRIDAY

I'm on a strange timeless time —
It's as though I could do this forever.
I'm reminded of crossing big oceans.
When I'm in the groove I could sail forever.
My friend Peter used to say that when you're at sea,
the only thing that matters is the weather;
and where I am now, the only thing that matters is Jade.
Not so much in a needy way, but more a vigilant one.
When you're at sea, the only way that it works
is to trust the other people to take care of the boat
— and help you while you sleep.

I know that J trusts me to keep her safe while she sleeps.
And I will, until my watch is over.
Janine told me days ago that the period that we're in now
— after talking is done but before her process is over,
is her (Janine's) favorite time.
I didn't understand.
She also described it as the mysterious time.
I get it now.
— I've spent hours sitting by her
listening to her breathe, rapt.
It's so clear to me
that even as her body is shutting down more + more,
her spirit is complete + totally intact.
It's like the intersection of church + state —
While it's clear
that there are two definite intersections between the two,
there are absolute laws that mandate separateness that,
in fact, define and celebrate their inherent differentness.

Everyone says don't guess,
but I'm guessing that she'll last the nite.
This afternoon, I wondered, but it's now 1am
+ she's gurgling some and blotching some
but somehow it feels like tonight isn't the night.
How much is me whistling in the dark —
I keep wondering how I'll be able to survive as a solo entity
after so long as J's partner.
I'll have to be a different me.
The experience of being her caregiver,
has changed me deeply + particularly this past week —
being forced to my knees from exhaustion
+ then held up by the love of my friends.
It could, if fostered, alter the course of the rest of my life.

Fear of change;
J is offering a real life example of non-voluntary change
done with grace + confidence.

Just last week she was lambastering me,
saying that I had to stop just assuming
that my way is automatically the best
+ learn to hear (at least) others' ideas as possibilities.
I so clearly remember considering being offended —
After ALLLLL I've done for you,
why do you have to spend our last hours criticizing?
— And then I realized
she was wanting to quick give me some last heartfelt advice
before she couldn't do it any more.

I've lived with an open heart
as we've lived together for the past week
and her body's useful life is ending —
I look into her eyes,
feel her heart pump and listen for her gurgling throat.
It seems that her last great lesson
must be that she and her body are not 1.
Her body is the little circus dog circling the ring
with a monkey riding its back,
the monkey in charge, the dog the carrier.
When the monkey is done with riding,
he simply hops off to do the next thing.
J's spirit is the monkey, her body the tired old dog.
Which leads to the question
if the monkey is so spry, where does it go?
Post-dog earthly life, what will that spirit do next?

There is a saying that if you don't learn this life's lesson,
you'll be condemned to that particular workbook
until you do.

It's like having to repeat fourth grade forever, or get it.
Maybe that's why J's body is hanging around for so long,
just to shove home her point.
Without good teachers, you'll never make it to the fifth.
Hanging around with all these women,
the analogues to giving birth are flying thick + fast:
You're not in charge.
It can hurt like hell when you're going through it.
After it's over it's hard, if not impossible,
to recite / rename the pieces that made up the whole.

This birthing / deathing thing that we're doing is both the
hardest + the most fulfilling that I've ever done.
It's a gift to me from J + to J from me.

Walking in Grace
is the easiest shorthand for the experience.

Working in and out of a time format.
I seldom wear a watch
and never know what day or time it is.
One of my cohorts
has taken to crossing off the days on the calendar,
not in a spirit of how long or short,
but a concession to the concept
that there is a world out there
with which we must keep at least loose contact
'til this process is done.

Random thoughts on the open-heart death at home:

It's hard.

It takes enough $ to be able to forget
about that important but worldly stuff for the duration.

You'd be an idiot to try + do it solo.

Having an in-house monkey
is not necessarily a help and can be a distraction
and musn't be allowed to interrupt
the most fulfilling thing I've done.

How can this compare to parallel shingle lines
or plum + straight wells?

Vanity, all is vanity.
Who said that?

SAT NITE

I had the sense that today J's spirit
was completely unaffected by what is going on in her body.
Beyond dark imaginings, there is a freedom
so enormous and comforting
that it makes even paradise seem constricting.
Our bedroom has become a transcendent space.
Time stopped here about a week ago.
I look at Jade and can't believe that being that skinny
is possible.
I had a spasm of sadness + loneliness + it just went away
in the same way that it was suddenly there,
it suddenly wasn't.

If thoughts come first, followed by emotion,
then the second thought can replace the first emotion.

Should we do a Scopolamine patch?

I have accepted the Janine / Islene premise
that the spirit + body are not essentially connected

+ I feel my role is to gently support the body
while waiting for the soul to finish up
whatever a soul needs to finish.
It takes as long as it takes.
It's a question of what finishes up first.
If the body is essentially the carrier-forward
of the essential spirit, then its work is done.
Remember the circus dog running around the ring
time after time with the monkey lightly,
seemingly effortlessly, being carried along.

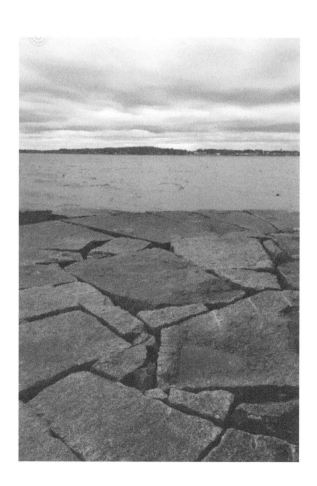

Life is amazing. So is Death.

The light is not extinguished as I take my last breath. . .
the age-old lamp with now shredded shade and wiring, is finally turned off
. . .at Dawn.

~Anonymous

Part Six

THE VALLEY
OF WONDERMENT

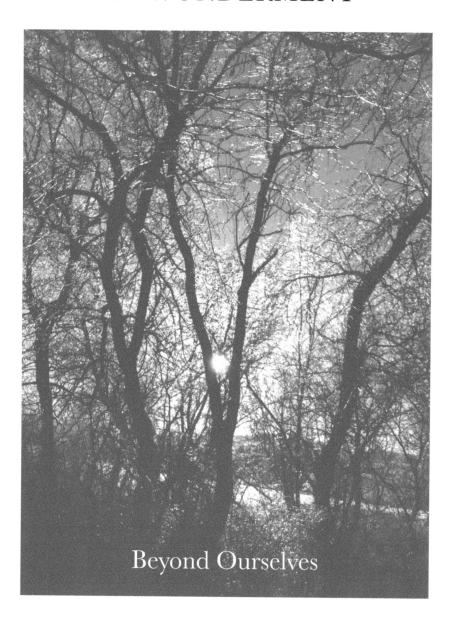

Beyond Ourselves

FIT ME

This is Jade's poem that she wrote four years before she died. Gordon shared it from her, along with pictures of them with smiles, their bodies and spirit together in their raw beauty. Jade had brown curly hair, *"And she's standing."*

Fit Me

I knew you before we met
As a puzzle piece knows its missing piece
By the you-shaped space in me.
My skate key
My allen wrench
You make it spin, fly, float, bounce
I come to a stop
Without you
I brake
I break
Without you
I love the high summer smell of your neck
Where it becomes the rest of you.
Sit here
Lean back on my legs
Let me sniff you
Fit me.

Jade slipped away to the land of feathers (chickens being her sign), around Thanksgiving. Little do I understand life, much less so death. Little do I know how Gordon is going to turn his next corner. I don't know even how I am going to turn my next corner. A dear friend wrote me today saying, in mid-winter, *"My spirit is very raw and tender. Sort of feels like I am dying from within."* There are no answers to give the despairing. Being there I hope is enough.

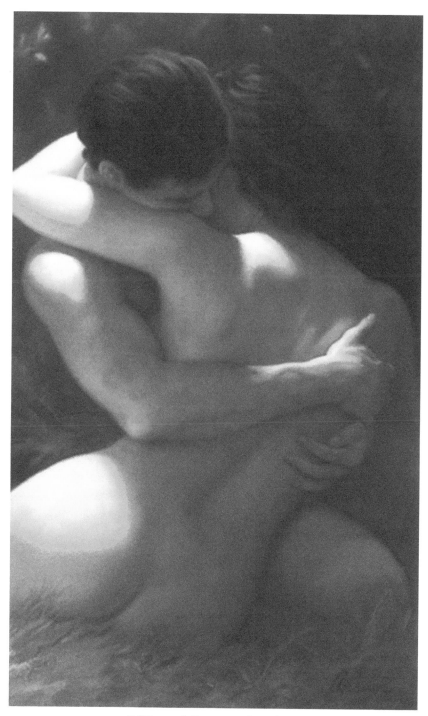

© "Carress" Courtesy of Mark Arian, proof.arianart.com

We all are despairing when we are.

"She is okay, that is all I know. Anyone who wants to preach to me about heaven can go shit in his hat. It might be true, but I am not hanging my hat on it. I hang my hat on only one little thing. I am not minimizing it, but it is only one thing. I refuse to generalize. She is okay, that is all I know."

"I wonder what Jade is doing right now as we talk," I mused.

"She may well have much more interesting things to think about," Gordon said. *"I don't really go by the hands-on-rails peering over and wondering how things are going. I am moving on; they can move on too."* We laughed.

Gordon and Jade had been advised by someone they trusted to get last rights before she died. *"I told her that could be a long assignment. Because Jade had not done confession since she was twelve. And she sinned a lot, trust me. But the priest came and said she was absolved of all her sins. I [Gordon] said, 'That's it? Then it's over? We're cool?' I am not sure he covered all the bases, from a theological point of view."*

When I went to visit my sister at Thanksgiving in California before Jade died, I told my sister that a patient would be dying any time, and that the patient had said her sign is: *"Chickens in an inappropriate place."* My sister and I agreed that the ones in her backyard did not count. Since they were in their "appropriate" place. When we walked out later in the morning, we smiled at her husband's incredulity that the gate was open, "impossibly so," he said. The chickens were running around the neighborhood. My sister and I winked at each other and had to agree that this counted as the sign we were looking for. Jade had died.

My sister and I talked about Sara's gravestone (the first person I nursed in true hospice care). The instantaneous peace I felt Sara sent me, on that day twenty years ago when I went to her gravestone to have a good cry, with the feeling that came instead, of immeasurable peace surrounding me at her rock. The dead are not as far away as it feels. Gordon spoke of the barrier between earthly living and whatever is after death, not unlike the wing of a dragonfly: Thin, slight, impossible to deny, no heavier, no darker, no less permeable.

Gordon said that when Jade died, her beloved and devoted caregiver of many years, Becky, and her brother, Sam, were on either side of her. *"That was okay with me. I was at her feet,"* Gordon said. *"I was rubbing her feet and her eyes were partly open. I don't know how much she could focus, but I stared right into her eyes. Everything we had been through came together, then she wasn't breathing. And I knew without any question at all that she was okay. I don't know where she went, but I knew she was okay, wherever she was."*

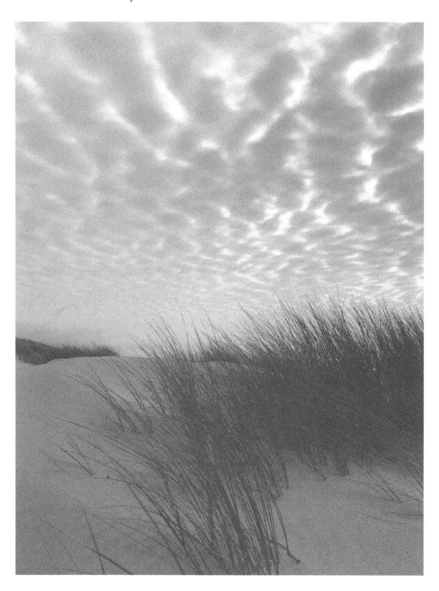

GOODBYE SOGIE

Gordon's shoelace was untied.
It was eighteen months after Jade had died.
He had an intimate friend in his life now who was a healer by profession.
She would become his wife in years to come. *"Life came along,"* he said.

Five years after saying goodbye to Jade, Gordon still mourned
the loss of a life where his needs had come secondary for decades
in what he called the wonderful package of his and Jade's marriage.
He had no romanticized or philosophized redemption of multiple sclerosis
in the context of what the disease stole from his marriage to Jade.

At 70-years-old, now re-married to the healer,
he has re-opened to himself in ways before he had been unable.
Richness and challenges rolled together
for a life he described as full, unimagined, in love.
The same Gordon re-opened to life, as we knew him with Jade.

Sogie, the monkey
who had entered Gordon and Jade's lives at a critical juncture,
had gone back to the training school when Jade had died.
Gordon was in a room now with Sogie in an attempt to briefly reunite.

Sogie had other things in mind.
*"She metaphorically and physically turned her back to me
and crossed her arms,"* Gordon described.
She peeked over her shoulder now and then,
trying very hard,
after eighteen months of her own grief and mourning,
to act like she didn't care that Gordon was now in the room.

Then, noticing Gordon's shoelace tantalizingly spilled on the floor,
her act started to sloppy.
She used to love to tie Gordon's shoes.

The ruin of a perfectly good pout and scowl,
the monkey went to tie Gordon's shoe.

And then, *oh heck,* jumped onto Gordon's lap.

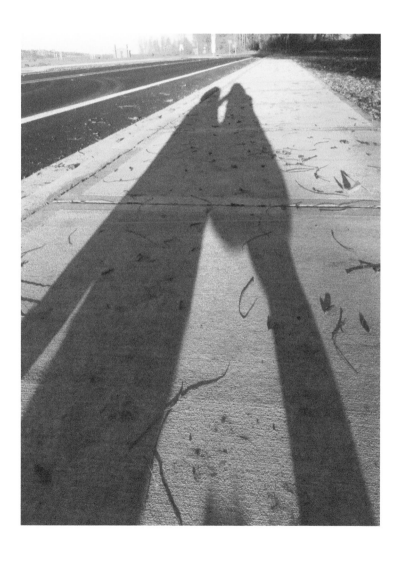

FIXING THINGS

Thomas died in his customary private and dignified way,
early Wednesday morning after reading his Monday morning paper,
asking for his nails and nose-hair to be trimmed
before his hospice "doctor" Therese was to arrive that same day,
then settling into a long, restful repose
while his family and beloved caregiver Rosemary held vigil
and kept him very comfortable.

Rosemary teased him for being in love with his "doctor" Therese,
the hospice nurse, and needing to look good for her.
And, now we know,
he wanted to look good for the ancestors he was preparing to visit.
He asked for potatoes to be cooked, and told his family
that he had done everything he wanted in his life, *"At least twice."*

He will no longer be calling his daughter every morning to check in —
Or at least not by telephone.
His family's postmortem choice of dress was the dark-green shirt
that he washed, pouring undissolved bleach into the colored load,
per his practice of taking care of it himself.
Large tan splotches on the shirt, and the torn hole from the weakened fabric. . .
The shirt, donned purposefully backward because he was bedfast,
adorned this resourceful, handsome, and solid life remembered.

He reportedly kept every fix-it-up item he needed in his garage,
but his sewing kit with huge needle eyelets, plus the ball of yarn
(its stitches seen darned in orange on the dark green shirt)
sat in reach on his hospice over-the-bed table.

The family thanked all the hospice *"angels."*

Thomas sends a wink, I am guessing, to his nurse Therese.
I imagine too that he is still busy fixing things.

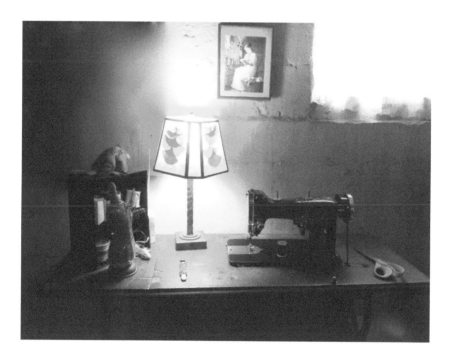

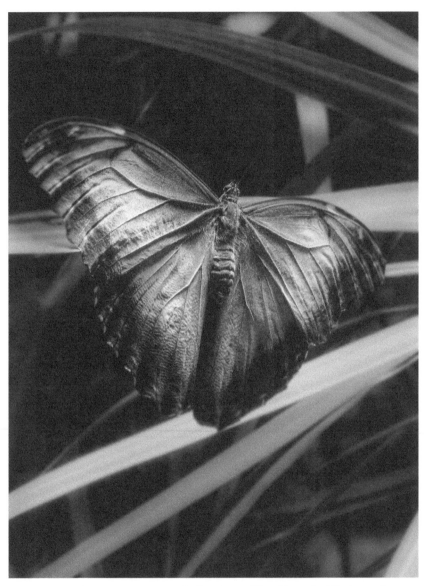

© Courtesy of SaraDowningPhotography.com

Nancy spoke of a butterfly/moth like this one visiting Siljoy just before passing. The same kind, she said, visited Siljoy's sister in Germany at the time of Siljoy's death.

NANCY'S LETTER

My beloved wife Siljoy Maurer left her physical body this past Friday afternoon July 20th. I was with her as she took her last breath. She passed with the dignity and grace that she lived her life. Hers was a peaceful passing.

Our community of family, friends, acquaintances, mentees and clients is vast and covers multiple continents. The very idea of organizing a physical get together for a celebration of her blessed life seems impractical and unattainable — our village is global. Siljoy and I discussed this numerous times and her response to this is "you will hear me in the wind and find me in the flowers" I also believe that part of her goodbye letter that she posted on June 18th was in direct response to her sense of what a service and closure look like. If you haven't read her goodbye letter I recommend you take a look. I re-read it yesterday and it is the essence of this remarkable woman. Scroll down her timeline and you'll find the letter.

It was a month ago that she wrote it. I can see her sitting in the cozy green recliner chair with her laptop in a deep focus telling her story and using every ounce of energy that she had. Once that was complete she progressed quickly towards her passing. It was a remarkable month. It was an incredibly painful loving privilege to accompany her to her exit from earth. It is a story that I would like to share, actually not just of this last month but of our journey from diagnosis to death. It is a blazing tribute to my wife and who she was.

Now it is up to all of us to practice what she lived which was living in integrity and engaging in the world with kindness.

She will find a way to continue to challenge each and everyone of us to do and be our very best in any given situation. I call it the Siljoy buzz.

I'll leave you with the wish that we blessed upon each other every day.....

"go forth and shine your light."

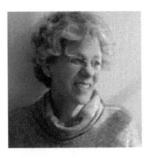

SILJOY'S LETTER

My final earthly days seem here ~ time to say Good-Bye...

Dear all, it is with peace, love and gratitude in my heart that I write these words. Some of You might have been wondering why I never posted again in the past 18 months.

On Thanksgiving 2017 I was almost killed in a red-light-runner situation. And — it was not my time yet. 4 weeks later, at Christmas, I was diagnosed with a very rare and hard to treat cancer. I have been calm and have done all within reason that held some promise of a chance to heal... My wife Nancy Barnett and I decided early on to continue to cherish every day together and not keep pursuing treatments when it seemed clear what was meant for me to happen... to focus on what would feel doable, manageable and kind enough and at the same time to continue to invite a miracle!

After having spent even a couple of months this winter in a German specialty clinic, to no avail, we stopped all treatments in March and I have been at home in hospice care since. I am surrounded by love and am so incredibly fortunate to have the best loving care in the world! We feel gifted by all this time we have had since my diagnosis (versus being killed in an accident and suddenly gone)... of course it has not been easy... and — we focus every day on what is good and beautiful, what we are grateful for and we begin every day with a little song we sing (even on chemotherapy or great pain days) :-)

It also allowed us the time to prepare and deal with a few more logistical pieces for after my death. Most importantly, I was given the time to say good-bye and help some of my Loved Ones as far as I can, to see beyond their pain and hardship after my transition to where there is only love and trusting that all happens how it is meant to happen! Naturally, at the same time, it is incredibly hard to leave Nancy and my families where we had hoped to have a lot more time together. And the truth is that we are all connected and needing to be together on the physical plane is ultimately just one piece of a deeper connection on a soul level.

For my Self, I have no fear — I have been in the "beyond our bodies" world before. And I KNOW that good and wonderful is awaiting me... I AM curious and wish from my heart that I will be able to be conscious enough during my dying process to experience my big transition fully...

Many asked me — why You? A holistic Mentor who always lived healthy and has always been incredibly strong? Well, internally, emotionally, spiritually, mentally I continue to be very strong, have been for the past 19 months, just my body is now very weak and struggling to properly function. And obviously I have not had any energy for being social. So I am mostly resting somewhere in our wonderful home, looking out the windows, observing the flowers and trees, the blue birds and pileated woodpeckers hatching their young or I am lying on a lounge chair outside in breeze... how can it get any better?! It is an interesting experience to become weaker by the day and observe my body fading away... I am giving her a lot of compassion and gratitude for having served me and lived with me for many years :-)

So back to the "why question" — I do believe in the benevolence of the Universe/ Divine which means that I implicitly TRUST that what is happening in one's life has PURPOSE, just, that often we can recognize that only in hindsight, right? It was also very hard for me to have to end all my mentoring relationships so very suddenly, not really who I am or what I would have chosen, if I had had a choice! When it became clear that despite admittedly poor chances to begin with, my body was not responding positively to ANY kind of treatments, it gave me/us the equally clear information that obviously, my life is meant to end soon.

And - I can easily accept that (as wonderful as it would have been to have many more good years with my Loved Ones)! And the beauty is that my life does feel complete, I feel complete! Since I was in my early twenties I always paid attention to not having any unfinished business and that is how I lived my adult life every day, so that any day could be a "best day for me to die"! It greatly helped me now, ultimately not even having much preliminary paperwork or such that needed doing and most importantly though that I truly feel at peace with everyone in my life... no old "stuff" to resolve — ALL is good!

And then there is also — MYSTERY! Do allow for mystery to be in your life... we cannot explain and understand all and I find the concept of accepting certain life experiences as MYSTERY incredibly comforting. I heard my Self say many times in the last weeks: it simply is! When You try that out and say it aloud — can You feel how grounding and calming that is... as the truth is always strengthening!

I am deeply grateful that I got to live several passions... immersing my self in integrative medicine and holistic thinking from early on in Europe... being one of the first official Mentors in the early 90's when no-one was talking about having a Mentor again, as it used to be throughout human existence until 100 years ago when community/family living fell apart.

...being one of the first 3 experts in the world to support and guide child-less people and being blessed with the most amazing success rate and having seen so many of "my" babies grow up on Facebook :-)

...following the legacy of my paternal ancestry and being a 9th generation gardener and tree-lover (my grandfather had the first professorship in the world for arborists and horticulturists in Berlin, Germany — it was created for him and has existed ever since)... having great joy working with rocks and stones and spending time in the wilderness.

...it is a little sad for me that I did not get to live my passion as a writer anymore — I always meant to write a couple of small books with information about my concept of the "Holistic Mobile" and its specific implications for how to change your life experience to a positive one... I know there are some things I taught that no-

one else has talked about yet... I trust that all my teachings over the years, whether in one-on-one mentoring, in the groups I led or in talks I gave will ripple out and somehow reach exactly the people for whom it would be good to learn about it...

I feel humbled to have been guided to consciously connect to the power of my ancestral/maternal side. A thousand-year-old lineage that I have drawn on for strength.

I want to appreciate each of You... with great love for my family, friends and beloved mentees and with respect for colleagues and other Facebook "friends."

Know that all is good and I am at peace... with great love.

~ Siljoy

And a last thought - when we make KINDNESS with Self and others our language of living, we always feel better...and we DO better in our world...one little step/ kindness at a time...!

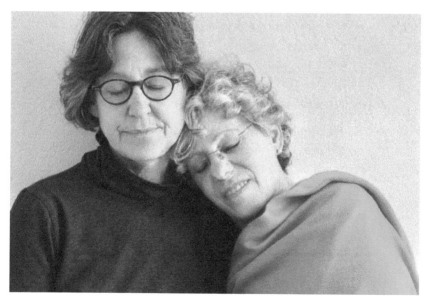

© Photo of Nancy & Siljoy by Nicole McConville

DRAGONFLY

White, silver, grey, touches of black, brown, more white, grey, silver.
The fine French braid elongated
in memory of the decades of Native American plus Swedish descendency
where being in touch with new dimensions
is ancestral knowledge, contrasting existential doubt.

"We are here because we are conscious.
We are not conscious because we are here," the son mused
as his mentor of grace and elegance, humanity and heart,
lay with hands overlapped.

His cell phone chimed,
cautiously requesting a lock of hair from her grandmother
who with advanced dementia
could not show recognition of the young woman,
then or ever again before tonight,
after the granddaughter dropped her habitual life
and moved to the Pacific Northwest
to help care for her grandmother.

I took the hair combs out of my hair and found the natural twirl
in the long braid shaped between notes of flute music playing on my phone.
The son cut it and laid it's soft curl carefully for the girl with the longing heart.
The Swede Native's remaining hair
was wrapped in the strand he first cut.
It brought her back to a sassy young girl of years past
with a short side pony-tail and a wink, I thought,
to the eyes that found themselves inadvertently resting on her natural beauty.

A dragonfly's wing's thickness between this world and the next,
Opaque from here, translucent in reverse.

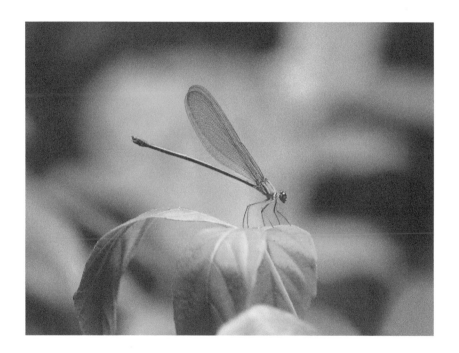

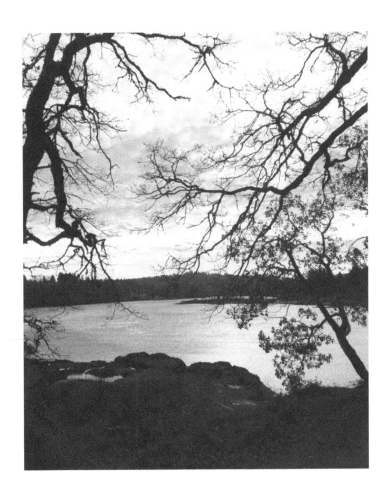

DEATH

Today I sat with death and
marveled at her beauty:
the thinning of her cheeks, the
slight in her brow, the
fix in her gaze, the
rustle of her breath, the
coolness of her skin, the
caress 'round her ears, the
tilting of her neck.

Today I sat with death and
her pale beauty and

I loved her.

~ Scott Wilson, M.Div., BCC

THE TO-DO LIST

Soothe the pain

Banish the nausea

Change the blood-soaked dressing

Search out the Root

Of the thing whose leaves Blacken life

Grasp, pull the Strength that was lost

Dust it off, Return it back as new

Roust the ensconced Disease

And if Time allows,

Turn life back to a Happier Day

So many things To Do,

But all you really asked,

Was that I stay and hold your hand

~ Rachel Houck, RN

Part Seven

THE VALLEY
OF TRUE POVERTY &
ABSOLUTE NOTHINGNESS

Less is More

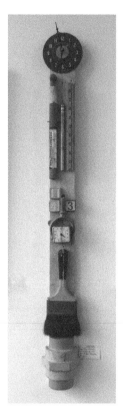

Clock I-43
© Ana Durley at River Gallery
Independence, OR

"Death is Nothing At All

Death is nothing at all

I have only slipped away into the next room

I am I and you are you

Whatever we were to each other

We are still

Call me by my own familiar name

Speak to me in the easy way you always used

Don't change your tone

Don't wear a forced air of solemnity or sorrow

Laugh as we always laughed

At the little jokes we enjoyed together

Play, smile, think of me, pray for me

Let my name be the household word that it always was

Say my name without effort

Without the ghost of a shadow in it

Life means all that it ever has

There is absolute unbroken continuity

What is death but this?

Why should I be out of mind

Because I am out of sight?

I am waiting for you for an interval

Somewhere very near

Just around the corner

All is well.

Nothing is past; nothing is lost

One brief moment and all will be as it was before

How we shall laugh at the trouble of parting when we meet again!"

~ Gordon's (Jade's husband's) slight alteration of Henry Scott-Holland's poem.

BROTHER

More stairs going deeper. No light. The landing at one level was caved in. Where did its depths go? I couldn't find the source water valve that my brother asked me to turn on for his newly planted trees. I was on vacation — no nursing this week.

The trees were not just on his property. His caring did not end at the surveyed marker. He was the one who taught me that we are stewards, not owners. I had to walk a couple of blocks past the graffiti and the torn-up sidewalk with the thriving dandelion scrounging its way through, past the Olneyville Tire corner-store with its ancient sign, past the curbside where the drivers didn't care if I was a pedestrian pulling a cart with four buckets of water to save a young tree in unexpectedly hot spring weather in Rhode Island.

The police car stayed on guard beneath the dirty underpass, his blue lights revolving. I wondered how many times he glanced at my novice navigation to the now updated property with a huge sign "YELLOW BRICK PATHWAYS, Community Employment Outreach". Or did he even care beyond the filth of the city?

The cathedral reached into the sky past the immediate exhaust odor and air of poverty and trash and abandonment. The magnolias and rhododendrons in bloom, climbing vines, and trees that had been planted and watered years back, had similar histories to my charges today. The arched windows and crafted edging, the stone and brick and slate that withstood weather, decades, and disappointment, held its own command, whether for the dead man last year found in the parking lot or the teenager lost in his headset, or me gazing at it and wondering how my brother could see past the fear and resistance and unawareness. How my brother could see potential in a forsaken corner that my daughter was told at her Ivy League school to never frequent Olneyville—that was the bad section of town, the dark part, unsafe.

I chuckled as I walked down deeper into the abyss of the antiquated church, with my cell phone flashlight my only guide. If my brother could own and restore this place, then I could turn the water on to save a few trees while he worked day and night shifts back-to-back helping lost souls find their real selves and discard the fabricated self image and diagnostic identity in exchange for their imagination and its creation of their real persona.

The hose didn't work very well. The source had frozen and was gushing water out the wall in a great spray, mostly missing the hose connection. So I was wasting water. Better than wasting trees, I could hear Todd say. Todd said he will have the trees spread all through the neighborhood before he dies.

Someone had left a towel on the bush, a dirty cloth bag lay strewn on the ground, a cigarette box and candy wrapper littered the small parking area. The buckets filled slowly. The water seeped in its own time around the roots of the sapling, some flowing into the street despite my efforts to keep it contained.

How far would the basement delve before the valve showed up? One room had a painting against the wall and a small chandelier hanging, mold and construction materials piled and discarded here and there. There was a huge shop with great tools disguised in darkness and dust. I had to call my brother for directions. Oh—I didn't think of passing the rows of stored pews after following a ramp I had missed, after circling through one dark room, another. Hitting the back wall of the back wall of the back wall and finding the electrical panels, was still not far enough. Another corner before the blue valve handle showed its face.

The awaited yellow brick pathway is for the new imaginations. A place to materialize skills and dreams, aptitude and connections. A dance school, a restaurant, a shop and more.

I am on the plane flying home to Oregon now. I am wearing a cream-colored dress and matching bracelet with the other well-dressed Americans on the flight. There is no dirt on overalls or black under the nails or dust in the hair and dirty sweat from restoration or landscaping. No broken faucets leaking or huge projects strewn in process. Well, of course there are different processes in process, but the plane TV screens did not show Olneyville or the basement that I did find my way into. No mold, no dark recesses of the despairing souls in the hospital where Todd takes on seventeen admissions in one night and talks to people without time cut-offs.

They could have been on a plane once and no one noticed their life was falling apart after they had spent it following the expectations and false structures, and when they had forgotten the dirt for their nails, and what cathedral was waiting to be found by them.

I didn't like going down in that darkness. I am not wimpy but it felt spooky. I remembered the day Todd hid in one of the rooms to catch a thief himself when the police were no help. My mind played games of wondering who might be down there now. A sense of being small and nobody wanted to penetrate into the heavy mildewy, seepingly cold air. Forgotten, lost, unseen. Decades and decades of history in the walls made my day seem a bit like a shallow breath—not even a deep refreshing single breath.

But Todd sees beyond all that, and so I rode his wagon. I went for the ride. The demons didn't like my chuckling. They were hungry for fear, doubt, shame, disillusionment, the defense of depression, inactivity, illusionary self-protection.

I chose my brother's protection instead. I'll ride that wagon.

"JUST DO IT" is written on the back of the t-shirt of the young woman on the plane at my right elbow as she sleeps with her head resting forward on the tray table. Someone else walking past the shadows to water the trees beyond our own properties.

Yellow Brick Pathways, Providence, RI

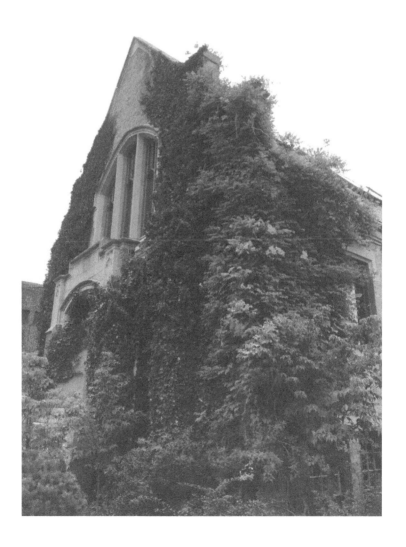

CHOOSING DEATH

The first "Super Moon" of 2014 (when the moon is closest to the earth) kept me working from 6am to 7am the next day. Full moons pull something powerful in their cycle, in births as deaths. Everything took its turn, as it does, with the help of the RN back-up, and the clinical supervisor admitting two patients after having worked all week.

It was nighttime in Independence, Oregon, one hour's drive from Portland. It is different here. There is more ease, less stressed rush and nerves in the culture. I am closer to the terrain I grew up in Mexico, closer to my daughters in Portland, speaking more Spanish to the many Mexicans who live here. I don't usually cry in my car any more. I belong here.

There are some big differences in hospice out West. One is that there is a plethora of Adult Foster Care Homes helping care for the ailing and the dying when they cannot be at home. These state-regulated family homes that have the connection that is difficult in nursing homes or larger facilities.

Another big change is that Physician Assisted Death is legal here, for people close to death already. It just became legal in Vermont, and Oregon doctors came to the first Vermont conference to help Vermont introduce itself to what is ahead. In Vermont, when I left there, neither doctors nor pharmacies wanted to enter the risk that is exposed in this venture. So it had not found its grounding there yet. In Oregon the practice is well established and, as Oregon physicians reported to Vermont, the legal cases evolving from unhappy families are at a stark minimum — mostly because the process is one of developing a deep understanding and relationship between doctor and patient, and opens an environment for trust.

My first confirmed Physician Assisted Death, after an anti-nausea medication and thousands of milligrams of the special kind of phenobarbital (given by family and / or a personal witness, not a hospice nurse, per regulation), was a woman who had polio disability since she was nineteen and had succeeded in living independently all her life. She was not going to give up this life-long victory, as she saw it, by becoming dependent in the death process.

I was nervous when called to "confirm" the death. (In Vermont, RN's "pronounce," in Oregon we "confirm" deaths.) For twenty-two years I have practiced the study of death in harmony with its nature, as it falls, letting go to what is, and the miracle of Mystery revealed, and not revealed, when released into the greater unknown. I was in foreign territory now: A patient had ended her life by choice and control.

I spent time in prayer before my visit asking to release my own expectations and judgments around dying, into the life of the family I was to meet, to learn from them about what I knew nothing.

On a side table at the entryway was a long list of tasks to be completed before the chosen time, on a piece of white cardboard half as tall as I am, in large, bold haphazard handwriting. Each item was crossed out. The house was completely bare. Every object, it seemed, had been allotted to its chosen place. A few name-tags lay scattered, forgotten, when the item had apparently been picked up.

The original plan was set for a date — preset a month later than this day — When the two sons were to visit. But the brother who attended instead, said that he was traveling in the area when his sister called him and told him that she was feeling the unwanted changes, and that it was time: Would he come and attend the death? "*Yes,*" he would, he told her.

He was calm when I walked in, alone with the body in the bareness, though in a separate room from her. He talked and engaged little. In fact his back was to me on the couch facing a blank wall. I wasn't positive at first that he was okay.

When a cousin came later saying, as a vet, that he had just used euthanasia for an animal, I could feel the foreignness of my situation. Then the brother and cousin spoke together of her life story, about her strength and her achievement of creating a living that was unintimidated by physical limitations.

They both spoke with pride and appreciation in their connection to a woman who knew her mind and did not let life daunt her at any stage, and lived to be 82-years-old.

.   .   .

When the full moon was high a month later, the "Super Moon" I alluded to, I was called to a different death that completely took me aback in its speed. The daughter said on the phone that her dad had woken up and asked if he could still take the PAD medicine — The one he had saved to end his life. He had not been able to swallow up to that point, and had been in and out of lucidity, but he spoke with clarity at this moment, she said, followed the exact protocol with the help of his beloved daughter, drank down the final drink of dissolved phenobarbital, slurping with energy at its last drops as it if were his favorite soda pop. It worked promptly. (It usually does, but not always.)

He was a respected scientist. A smart brain, a man who trusted knowledge and orchestration, and maybe knew less of the insecurity of facing the unknown when learning new arenas late in life. His daughter said he denied spiritual association.

When I met him on Friday, it took a lot of Haldol to get him out of his head, and relaxed. He was tense, agitated, confused. His daughter said that he was watching his own process, thinking it through, analyzing it, weighing it, and not understanding it. At that time, despite his struggling, he did not want the final medication that he had carefully stored for the right time.

When he finally slept deeply on Friday night, he spent the next day in what I call the world of connection between earth and spirits or spiritual world. He spoke freely to people who had died, made the associations that only the dying seem to know how to do, and had leaped into the world that just yesterday he was resisting with gusto. (The gift of the right therapies at the right dose, releases the hospice patient to do the work they need to do.)

Through tears of incredulity, the daughter walked me up the stairs to his apartment, telling me about how he woke from a deep sleep, asked how long he had been *"like this"*, said he wanted to walk to the bathroom to pee (up to then he had not been able to walk), and when achieved, said, *"Do you think I can still take the medicine?"* He was ready. And his family was ready to meet him there.

The daughter afterward said she was so proud of him. She had found some notes delineating his desires just as they came to be: Who was to be there and how it was to be done. That is how it happened. He had lived a life of command and scrutiny and determination. He died with command and scrutiny and his determination, at peace.

"That was my dad," Penelope said, unaware of her own exhaustion from the last days, with the Moon so bright in the sky that we both felt we were in a different world for the night.

I marked it, reminding myself that it isn't a different world; it is our world, in all its unfolding dimensions.

HE SAID

"It's the questions that matter,

we chase the world for answers
but the questions are what are important

for there are no answers
none,
zero,
zilch.

There are no answers.

I have these religious people
come to my door
and tell me what to believe
but when I sit them down
and talk with them
they're terrified
they hold to their answers
like a child holding a teddy bear
in the middle of a storm

because there are no answers,
there are no answers, but
there are questions

we must live into the questions.

And it's not that someday
when we die
we will get the answers
we won't

because there are no answers
but we will come to a place
where we no longer need the answers
because we will no longer need the questions
where we can just be

and won't that just be
wonderful."

~ Scott Wilson, M.Div., BCC

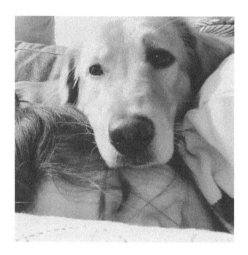

GRACE

She was crying out in pain. Retention of urine it appeared. I had to catheterize her quickly. Done. Yes, the retained yellow fluid flowed steadily. I ran to the bathroom to empty one drainage bag for another. "Urine never comes out this fast," I said to myself. No wonder the bladder had been hurting so. The second bag started to fill as fast. This time it was bright red. The blood filled the next bag in no time before I blocked off the clamp.

Only puncturing a primary artery could drop blood this fast. Even then it was impossibly rapid. With a urinary catheterization? She could not survive this amount of blood-loss in her end-of-life condition. Then in seconds everything was over. She was gone. I had killed her. A flash of all lost went before me.

I sat up in my bed breathing hard, sweating, my head racing. I had only a few hours of sleep this holiday weekend but I didn't dare close my eyes for fear of facing the nightmare again.

A few hours earlier I had arrived at a home where Tom had a seizure because he would regularly refuse his anti-seizure medications and has epilepsy. In his fierce independence and quest for power to control his world, he refused to get up off the floor or be touched for 30 hours after yesterday's seizure. His brother, the person to whom he was closest, had spent hours with him that day, in two visits, and had left with the patient still on the floor, angry and ready to hit anyone who got close.

After his brother had left, Tom had decided to get up on his own, went to the bathroom, dress in warmer clothes, and busied himself in his room. (His brother had melted him even if it did not look like it at the time.) The nurse (myself) was announced. *"Go away,"* he bellowed.

I sat down with the owner and caregiver in the living room and told them that my primary task purpose today was to get him to take his anti-seizure medicines so we could avoid these episodes. *"Good luck,"* said the owner. *"I'll wager you $1.00 it won't happen."* I laughed. The owner had had a long couple of days.

I asked to sit quietly for a while. The owner said to wave a hand to him when I was ready so he could be nearby to help keep me safe. His mother, also a caregiver in the home, had gotten hit in the jaw by Tom recently.

"Has he eaten anything during this time?" I asked. *"Nothing."* "Will you give me something he likes to eat? And his medication?" I had my tray in hand with his favorite cookie. I sat longer in silence to let go all distractions from what the patient showed he needed, and then walked to the door and knocked. *"Just a minute,"* he said. "Okay," I answered.

I waited a minute. Two. Four. Five. I stood at the door and listened to his feet shuffling to get a clue if he had forgotten me or was trying to complete a task before letting me in. He was known to be a busy man. I knew that pushing him before building any rapport would take us backward. Should I say anything? Ten minutes. Should I knock again? The sounds were of some focused task. Did he know I was standing there? How much had his many seizures caused brain damage and how cognizant was he right now? Twelve minutes. (I wasn't actually counting, but the time kept ticking on.)

Then he spoke. *"Where is my dollar bill?"* I thought I had misheard him, so I asked him to repeat himself, knowing it was important to know exactly what he had said (even if it was risky because any request to repeat himself could add to irritation and feeling not understood). *"My dollar bill!"*

"Oh," I said. "I think it is out here. Let me look." Fortunately the owner had a dollar bill in his pocket. I am glad he meant his wager, I said to myself. I knocked and walked straight in without waiting for further invitation. "I found it, here," I said handing him the money. He looked surprised to see the bill.

"I also brought you a cookie and your medicine." I was upfront about the medication for trust, so he did not think I was hiding it with a cookie. "Would you like a bite?"

"No."

"Okay," I said. "It sounds like you had a really hard day; I am sorry."

"Yea, it was a hard day."

"Tom, I want you to take this anti-seizure medication. It is very important to keep you from having as awful a day as you have had today." I spoke with a firmness that a weary person might bend to.

"Okay," he said. He took the liquid he hated the taste of.

"This is the pill that you should also take." I did not hand him the medicine. I held the tray still and he reached for himself. "May I help you finish pulling up your trousers?"

"No."

"Okay. If there is anything else I can help you with I would be glad to."

"No."

"Okay. Well it is good to see you. We are nearby if you need anything." I left the room, leaving the cookie and tray on his table. *"You could have cleaned up the mess you made on the floor,"* I heard from inside the room.

I went back in. He had his cookie in his hand and had taken a bite. There was feces on the floor. This was a fastidious man and he wanted it cleaned it up, but I figured blaming me felt more discreet.

"I am sorry," I said. "I will be glad to clean it up." I took my time cleaning. He sat in his recliner. He pointed to a painting on his wall and said something about it. He said it was his grandfather's. I asked him about his grandfather. We chatted. His arm was not in his sweatshirt sleeve. "That sleeve looks like it is off-kilter."

"Yea, something is wrong here."

"Let's see, maybe I can help." He was more comfortable with is arm in the sleeve.

Then, pointing to some soiling on his hand, allowed me to clean it up. I asked him if I could sit on his bed. He said yes. We talked about his bad day, his feeling stiff, his brother whom he had forgotten had visited, casual conversation. He let me make his bed invitingly and I told him I was glad to be able to visit with him. We shook hands, and I reminded him that we were close if he needed anything. He said *"Thank-you."*

The caregivers and I made some new plans for regularity of taking his medications, reducing the number of pills with prioritization, using a spoonful of grape juice concentrate for maximum flavor and minimum volume to mask bitterness, plus more.

Just before this visit, my colleague had sent me to see someone else: "I am glad you are going. I don't know what I would do about someone's face turning black. You are so much more experienced."

"The most important way I am different with experience," I mused, "is that when I arrive at a door and am clueless as to either what I am going to find or how I am going to help with the problem identified, I don't panic any more, and I wait... I wait for as long at it takes, until the clues show up."

So far we haven't killed anyone.

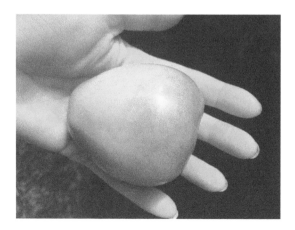

LOOK AT IT

"He said a lot of things," his son lamented.

"I don't know if I did well by him.

I don't know if he was comfortable, I don't know much."

As his nurse, I came to confirm the death

of his father's stiff body in the adjustable bed.

His mother had died six weeks prior.

"This sounds a little corny," he said,

"But our mother died on the full moon – A sliver short of it.

Our father died on a new moon – A sliver short of it.

Together, the two make a complete full moon.

Or a complete new moon, however you look at it."

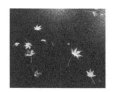

To teach is to learn.
To learn is to work.
To work is to serve.
To serve is to love.
To love is to sacrifice.
To sacrifice is to die.
To die is to live.
To live is to strive.
To strive is to rise above all earthly limitations
and enter the eternal realms.

~ Abdú-l'Bahá

FEROCITY

A fancy resort.
Two lovers who still were still lovers after decades of making a life together.

They thought he was going to be the one to die first.
Oxygen dependent, multiple diseases piled on top of the last.
The EMT's were there for him, far away from the city, often on a monthly basis.
But it was she who came into hospice. Unsuspected lung cancer.

"My parents waited until they retired
to do all the special fun they wanted to do together."
But instead, illness and death came with retirement.
"Before my mom died she told us to not wait."

"We have had camp fires, many camp fires," he interrupted,
both of them storytelling, laughing, smiling.
He said it more than twice. She did most of the talking.

At the resort they wanted the place to themselves.
"We were exhausted, and we needed it," she said.
It was an elite private place with a long driveway from the main road to the inn.
They parked at the end of the driveway,
scheming how to scare the weekend guests away.
They drew up all their enthusiasm for each car arriving to a weekend at the inn.
"Come on in! Come on in! We have a rock'n band, lots of beer!!
It will be a hoot'n party!"

Why did each car turn around and go away?
Too rowdy for the conservative clientele?
Too bad. The couple had the place to themselves that night.

"We needed it," she repeated. Only stealthy glee, not a mark of shame.

She then wanted to see a friend in Arizona. And ride a motorbike again.
She did so.

Finally, pneumonia and a pleural effusion flew her home from Arizona
on emergency medical transport so she could die at home.
First my nurse colleague, then I, spent much of last night with her
and her husband, helping her transform her fierceness
into the presence and quieting that death requires.

Not on her watch, her body and spirit said,
but the clock (that was not on the wall)
and her ferocity that thought it did not like the face of death,
did witness her discovery of release.

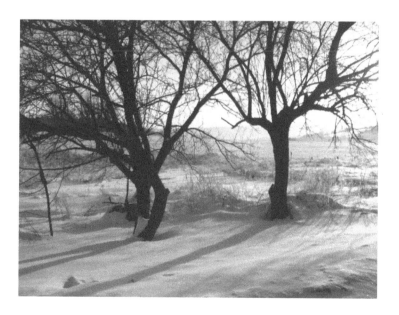

MY OWL

A wide expanse of wings.
Cream-speckled feathers on a robust body.
How many times have I driven the countryside East and West
taking in companioning hawks, ospreys, owls, ravens, eagles
in the celestial expanse.

How could there be seven different rainbows — with coupled ones
around new corners — on creamed clouds in one perfect evening?
A sign of pure joy in all valleys of this life.

Tonight an impossible catheterization that was successful by grace.
Pain, fear facing death… Then ease.
The wife called in the morning to say the ease was a first in days.
I could hear her breathe deeply unlike like last night in the tension.

My colleague friend called telling me she (the nurse) had choked.
Her daughter saved her with the Heimlich.

My lover felt far away in the still of the night
without his arm around me to even-out the unsettledness of life.

How then the thud against my car?
Too late before I had time to see the flying bird of prey.
Monte my dog companion also thudding forward with my hard braking,
the catheter bag falling over him.
How the huge bird falling onto the car hood,
then wobbling with lame wing into the bushes to hide?
How more wounds and nearness to death on a silent night?

An open slate to its signs of meaning on the waves of life, my brother said.

I know now what it means for me, though it took me until today
to see it beyond the tears and wrench in my heart.

Death is not what it is hyped.
Nor is it only heavenly and all redeemed.

The owl calls us.

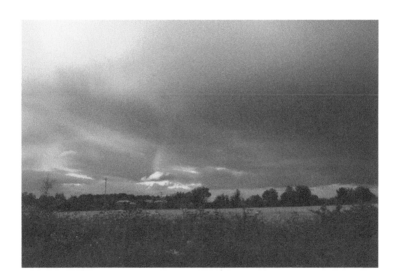

PostScript

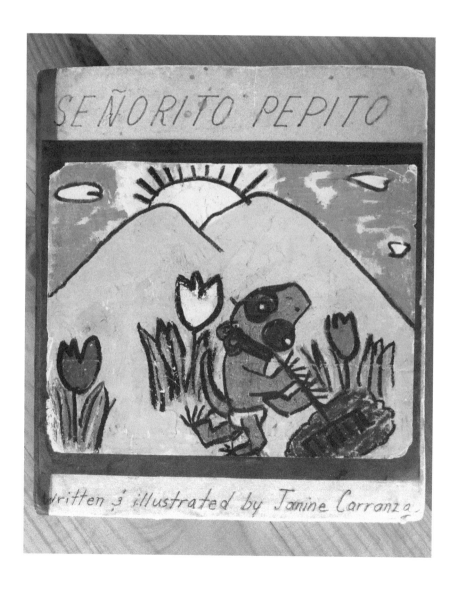

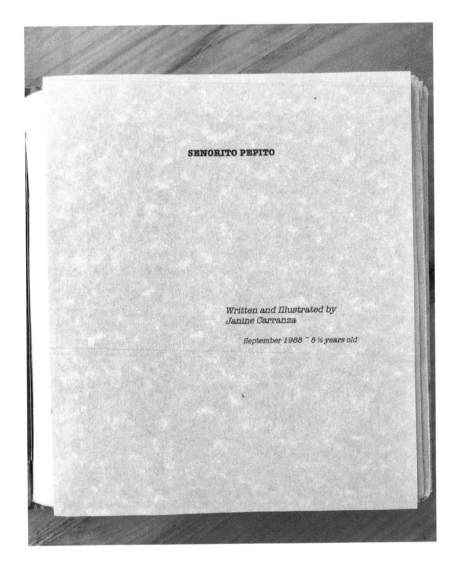

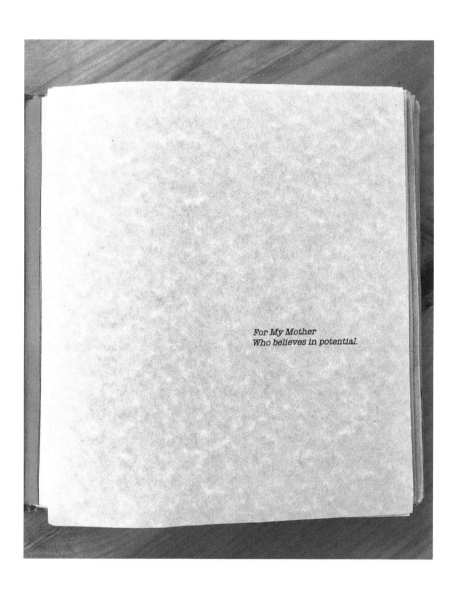

For My Mother
Who believes in potential.

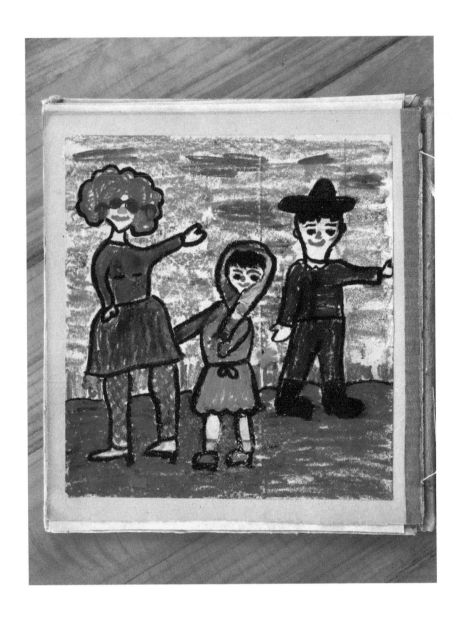

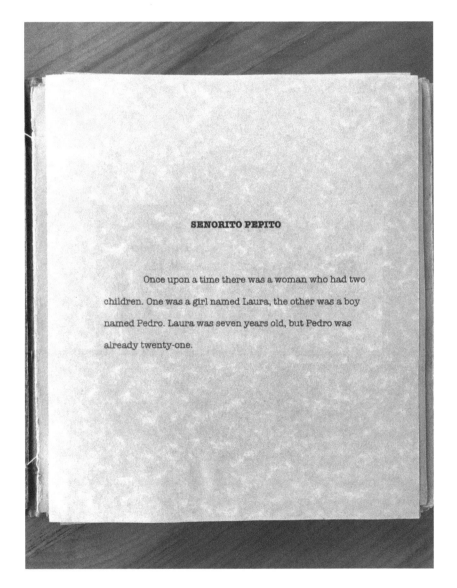

SENORITO PEPITO

Once upon a time there was a woman who had two children. One was a girl named Laura, the other was a boy named Pedro. Laura was seven years old, but Pedro was already twenty-one.

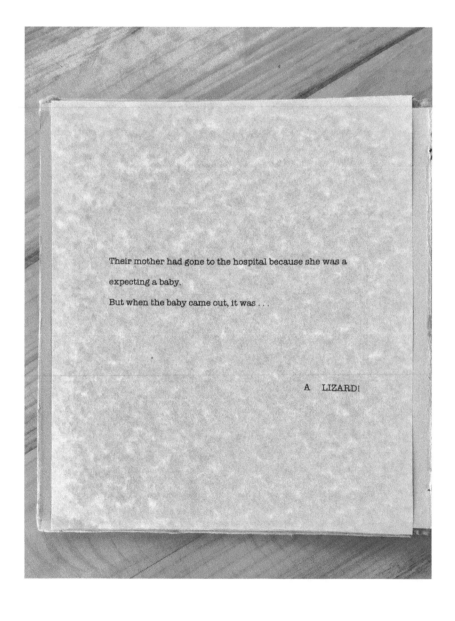

Their mother had gone to the hospital because she was a

expecting a baby.

But when the baby came out, it was . . .

A   LIZARD!

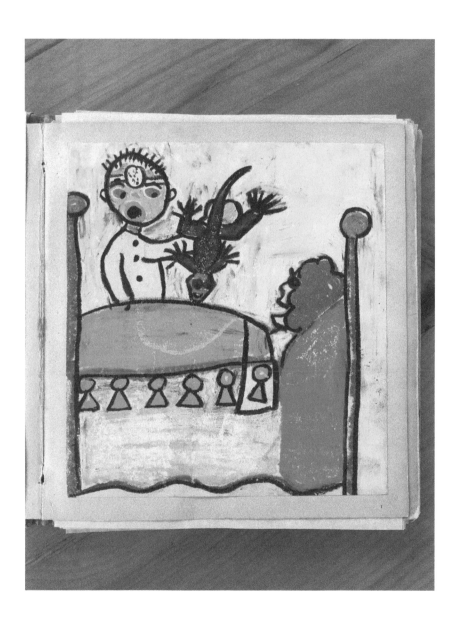

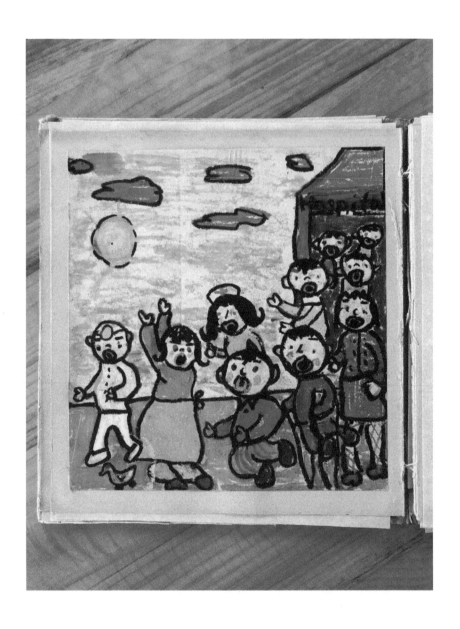

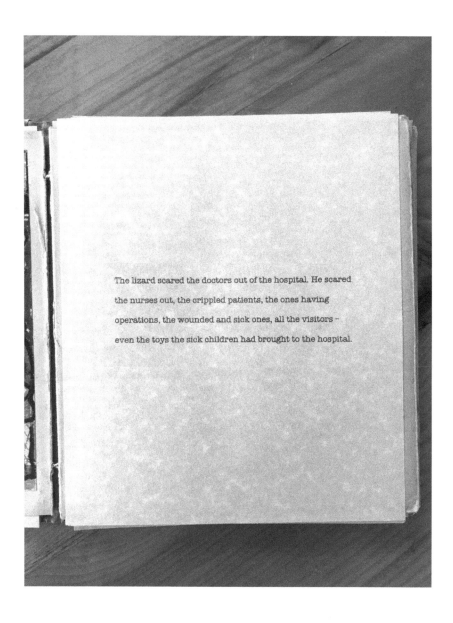

The lizard scared the doctors out of the hospital. He scared the nurses out, the crippled patients, the ones having operations, the wounded and sick ones, all the visitors – even the toys the sick children had brought to the hospital.

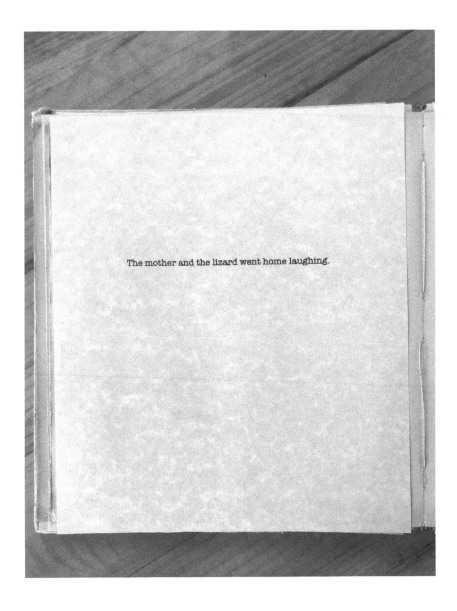

The mother and the lizard went home laughing.

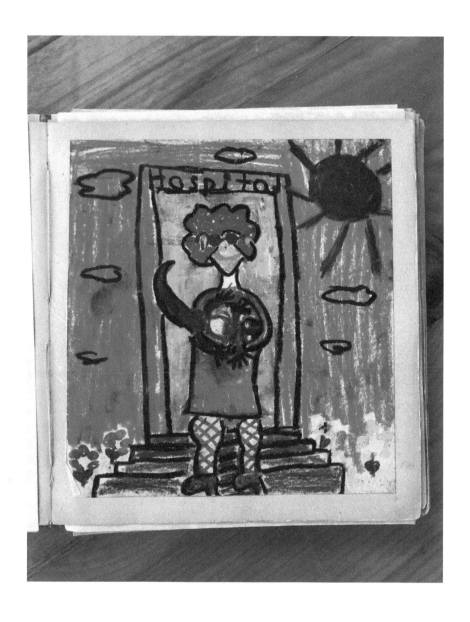

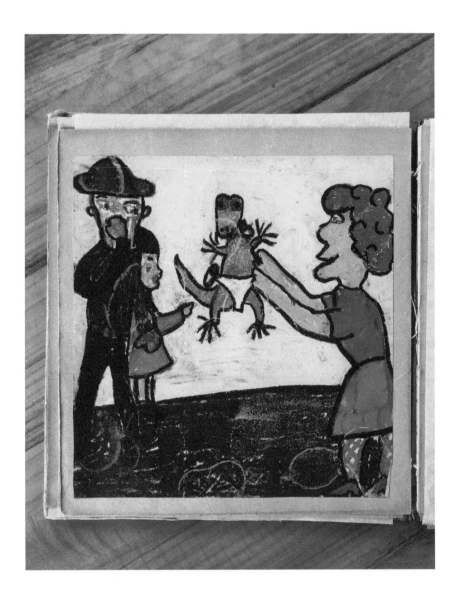

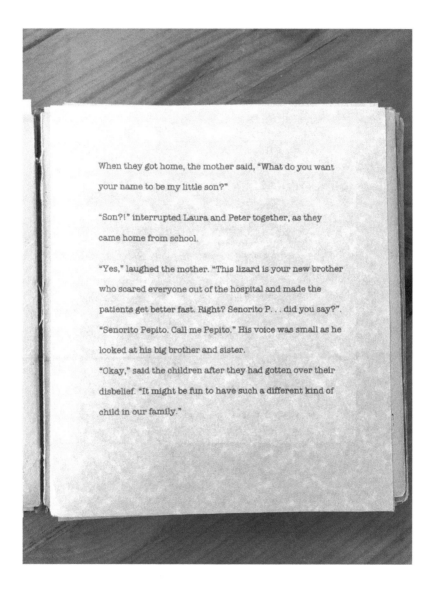

When they got home, the mother said, "What do you want your name to be my little son?"

"Son?!" interrupted Laura and Peter together, as they came home from school.

"Yes," laughed the mother. "This lizard is your new brother who scared everyone out of the hospital and made the patients get better fast. Right? Senorito P. . . did you say?".

"Senorito Pepito. Call me Pepito." His voice was small as he looked at his big brother and sister.

"Okay," said the children after they had gotten over their disbelief. "It might be fun to have such a different kind of child in our family."

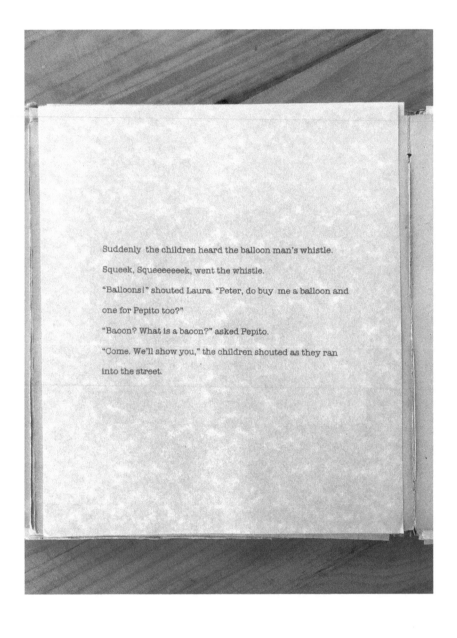

Suddenly the children heard the balloon man's whistle.

Squeek, Squeeeeeeek, went the whistle.

"Balloons!" shouted Laura. "Peter, do buy me a balloon and

one for Pepito too?"

"Baoon? What is a baoon?" asked Pepito.

"Come. We'll show you," the children shouted as they ran

into the street.

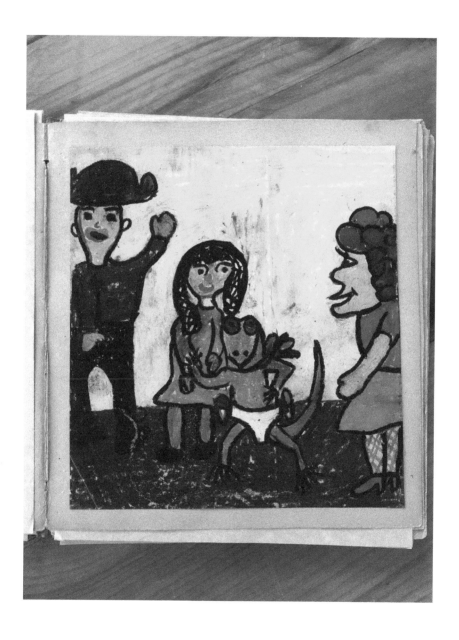

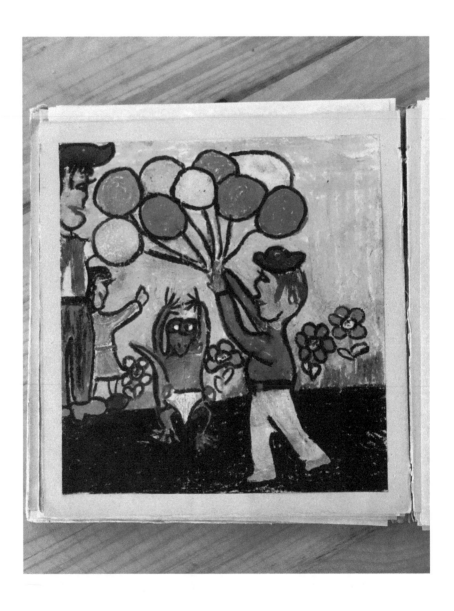

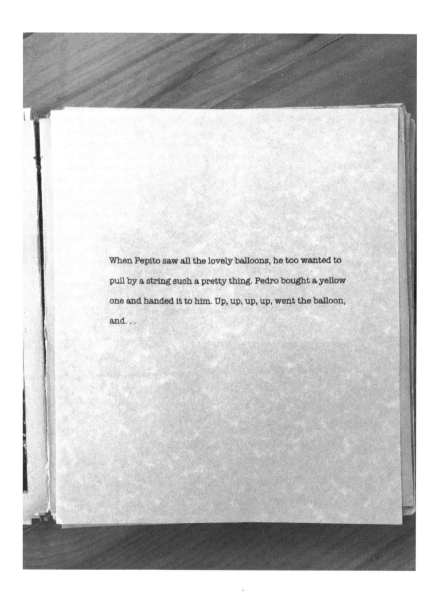

When Pepito saw all the lovely balloons, he too wanted to pull by a string such a pretty thing. Pedro bought a yellow one and handed it to him. Up, up, up, up, went the balloon, and. . .

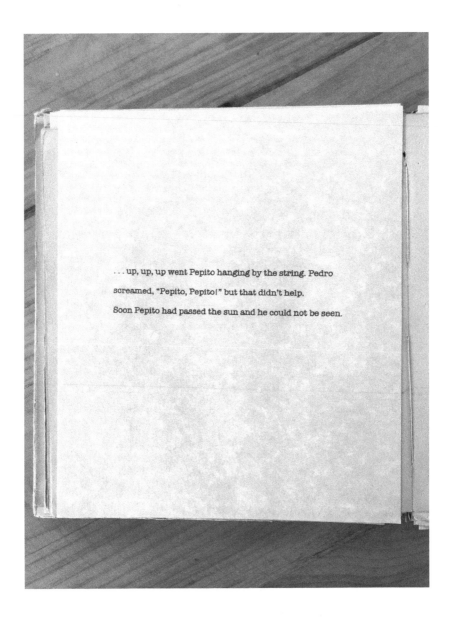

...up, up, up went Pepito hanging by the string. Pedro screamed, "Pepito, Pepito!" but that didn't help.

Soon Pepito had passed the sun and he could not be seen.

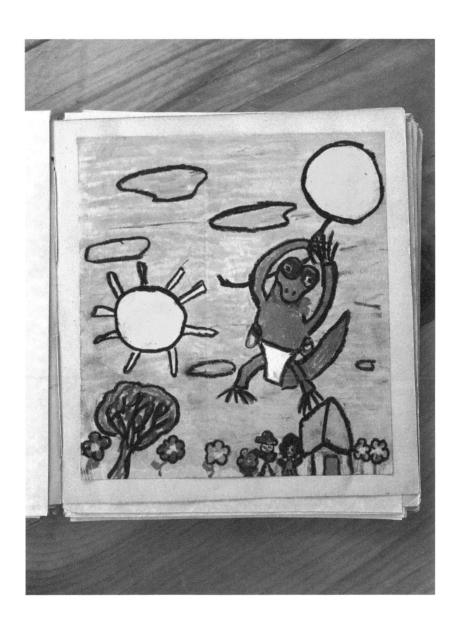

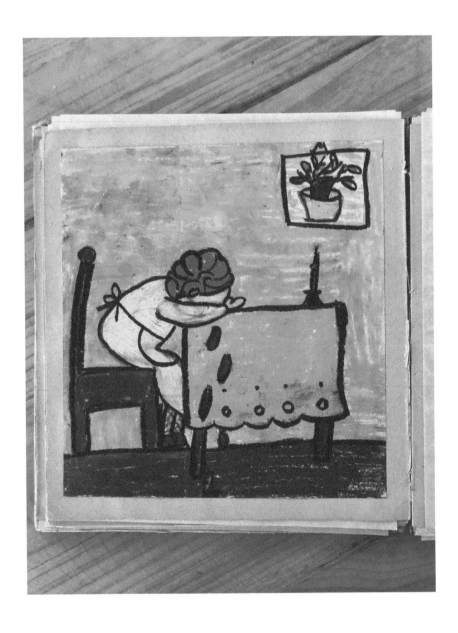

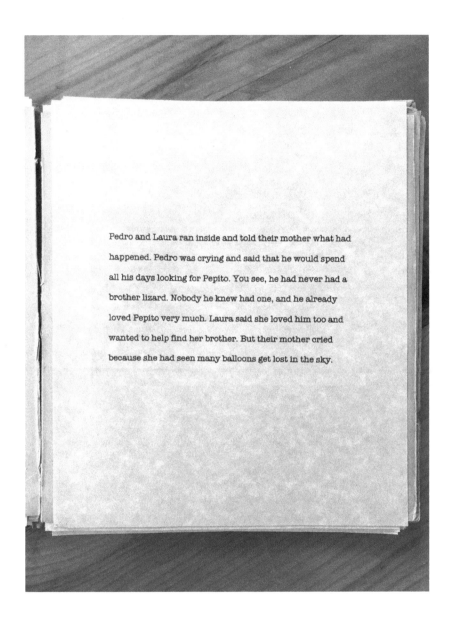

Pedro and Laura ran inside and told their mother what had happened. Pedro was crying and said that he would spend all his days looking for Pepito. You see, he had never had a brother lizard. Nobody he knew had one, and he already loved Pepito very much. Laura said she loved him too and wanted to help find her brother. But their mother cried because she had seen many balloons get lost in the sky.

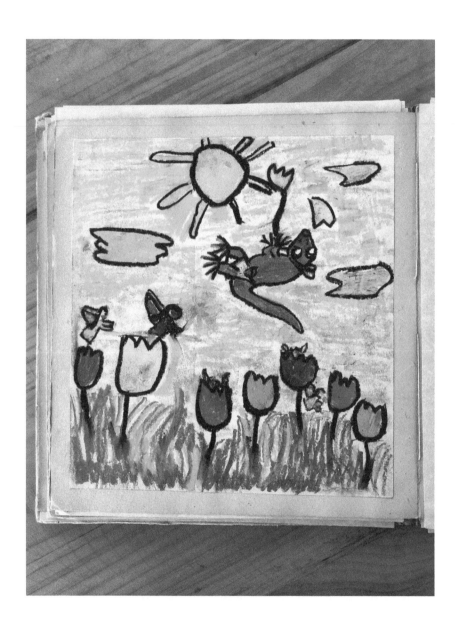

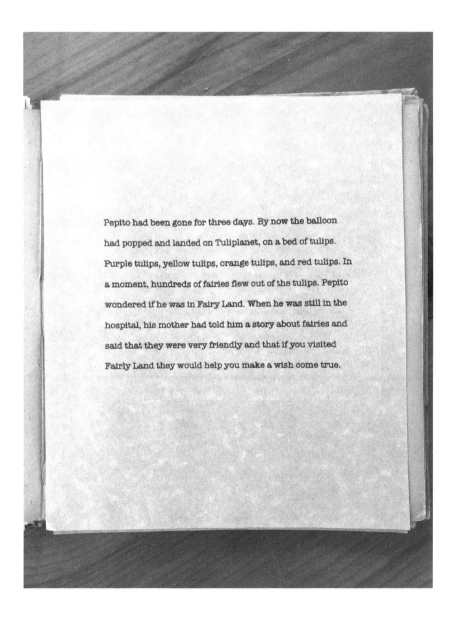

Pepito had been gone for three days. By now the balloon had popped and landed on Tuliplanet, on a bed of tulips. Purple tulips, yellow tulips, orange tulips, and red tulips. In a moment, hundreds of fairies flew out of the tulips. Pepito wondered if he was in Fairy Land. When he was still in the hospital, his mother had told him a story about fairies and said that they were very friendly and that if you visited Fairly Land they would help you make a wish come true.

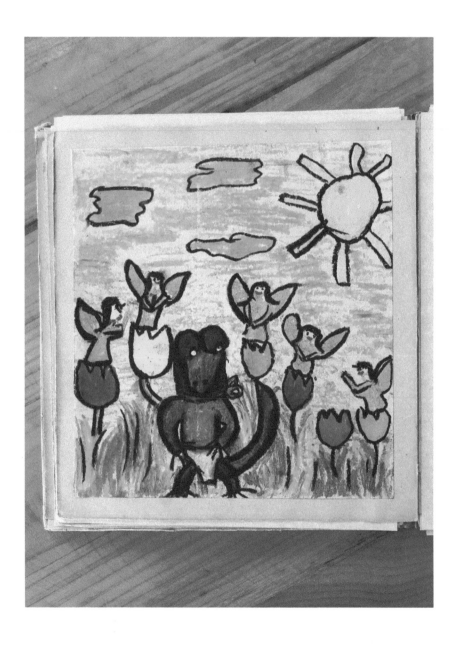

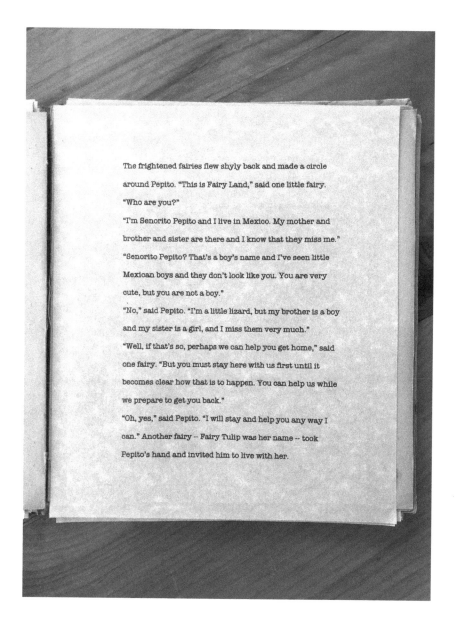

The frightened fairies flew shyly back and made a circle around Pepito. "This is Fairy Land," said one little fairy. "Who are you?"

"I'm Senorito Pepito and I live in Mexico. My mother and brother and sister are there and I know that they miss me."

"Senorito Pepito? That's a boy's name and I've seen little Mexican boys and they don't look like you. You are very cute, but you are not a boy."

"No," said Pepito. "I'm a little lizard, but my brother is a boy and my sister is a girl, and I miss them very much."

"Well, if that's so, perhaps we can help you get home," said one fairy. "But you must stay here with us first until it becomes clear how that is to happen. You can help us while we prepare to get you back."

"Oh, yes," said Pepito. "I will stay and help you any way I can." Another fairy -- Fairy Tulip was her name -- took Pepito's hand and invited him to live with her.

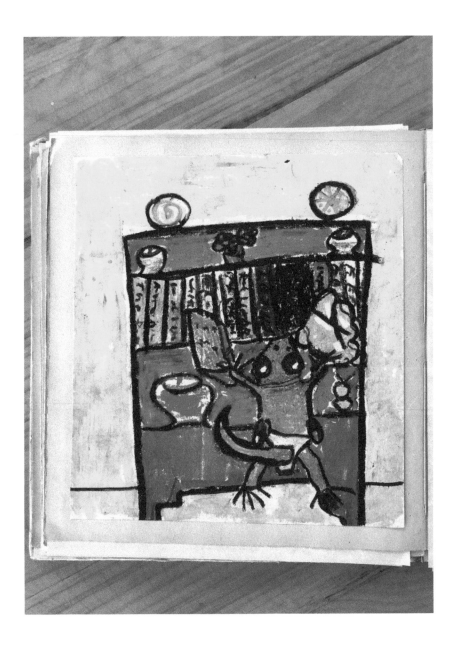

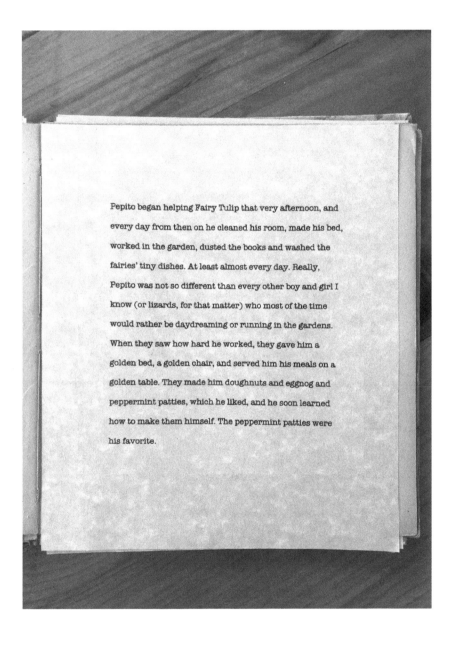

Pepito began helping Fairy Tulip that very afternoon, and every day from then on he cleaned his room, made his bed, worked in the garden, dusted the books and washed the fairies' tiny dishes. At least almost every day. Really, Pepito was not so different than every other boy and girl I know (or lizards, for that matter) who most of the time would rather be daydreaming or running in the gardens. When they saw how hard he worked, they gave him a golden bed, a golden chair, and served him his meals on a golden table. They made him doughnuts and eggnog and peppermint patties, which he liked, and he soon learned how to make them himself. The peppermint patties were his favorite.

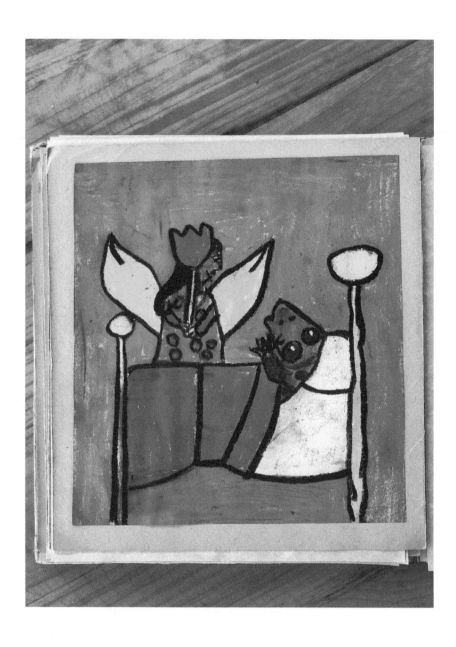

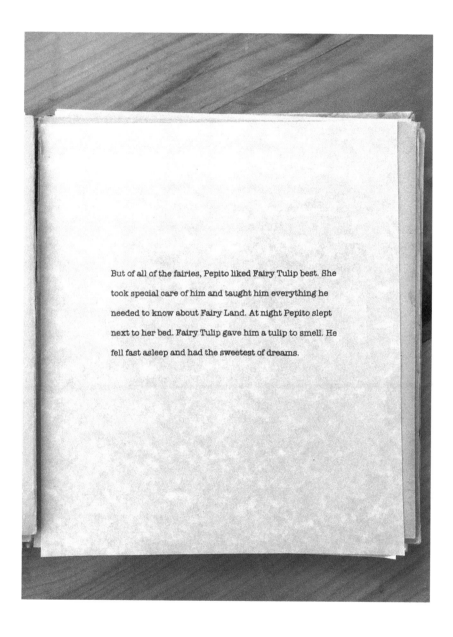

But of all of the fairies, Pepito liked Fairy Tulip best. She took special care of him and taught him everything he needed to know about Fairy Land. At night Pepito slept next to her bed. Fairy Tulip gave him a tulip to smell. He fell fast asleep and had the sweetest of dreams.

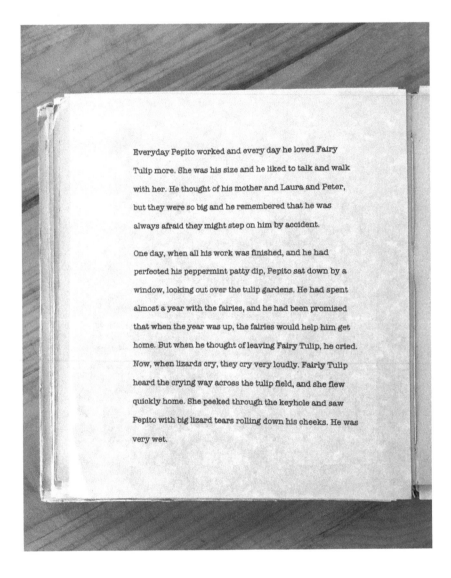

Everyday Pepito worked and every day he loved Fairy Tulip more. She was his size and he liked to talk and walk with her. He thought of his mother and Laura and Peter, but they were so big and he remembered that he was always afraid they might step on him by accident.

One day, when all his work was finished, and he had perfected his peppermint patty dip, Pepito sat down by a window, looking out over the tulip gardens. He had spent almost a year with the fairies, and he had been promised that when the year was up, the fairies would help him get home. But when he thought of leaving Fairy Tulip, he cried. Now, when lizards cry, they cry very loudly. Fairly Tulip heard the crying way across the tulip field, and she flew quickly home. She peeked through the keyhole and saw Pepito with big lizard tears rolling down his cheeks. He was very wet.

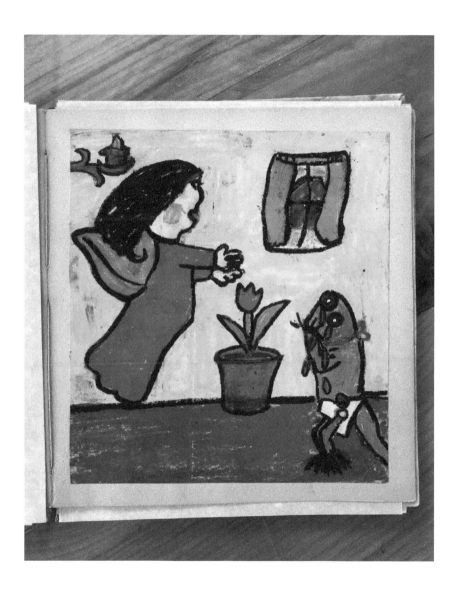

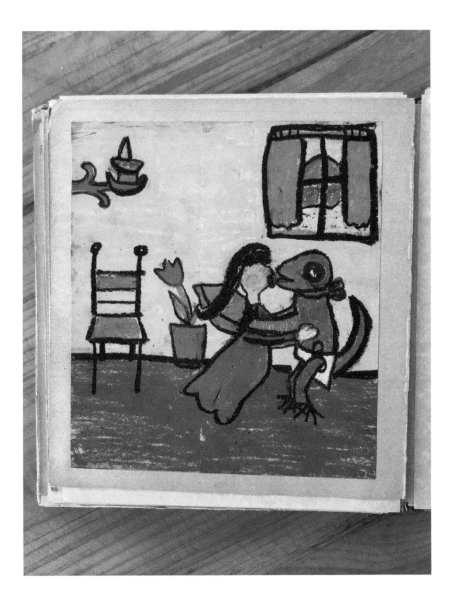

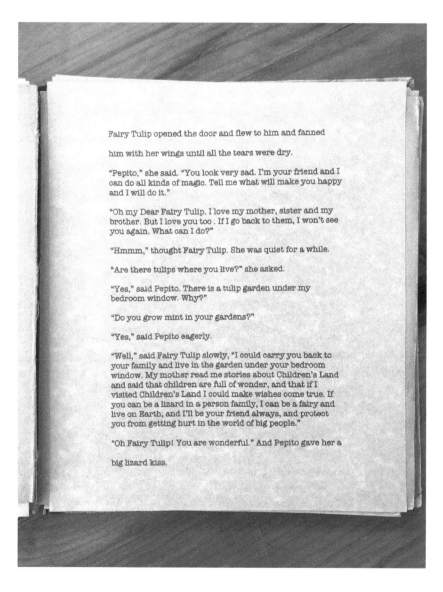

Fairy Tulip opened the door and flew to him and fanned

him with her wings until all the tears were dry.

"Pepito," she said. "You look very sad. I'm your friend and I can do all kinds of magic. Tell me what will make you happy and I will do it."

"Oh my Dear Fairy Tulip. I love my mother, sister and my brother. But I love you too . If I go back to them, I won't see you again. What can I do?"

"Hmmm," thought Fairy Tulip. She was quiet for a while.

"Are there tulips where you live?" she asked.

"Yes," said Pepito. There is a tulip garden under my bedroom window. Why?"

"Do you grow mint in your gardens?"

"Yes," said Pepito eagerly.

"Well," said Fairy Tulip slowly, "I could carry you back to your family and live in the garden under your bedroom window. My mother read me stories about Children's Land and said that children are full of wonder, and that if I visited Children's Land I could make wishes come true. If you can be a lizard in a person family, I can be a fairy and live on Earth, and I'll be your friend always, and protect you from getting hurt in the world of big people."

"Oh Fairy Tulip! You are wonderful." And Pepito gave her a

big lizard kiss.

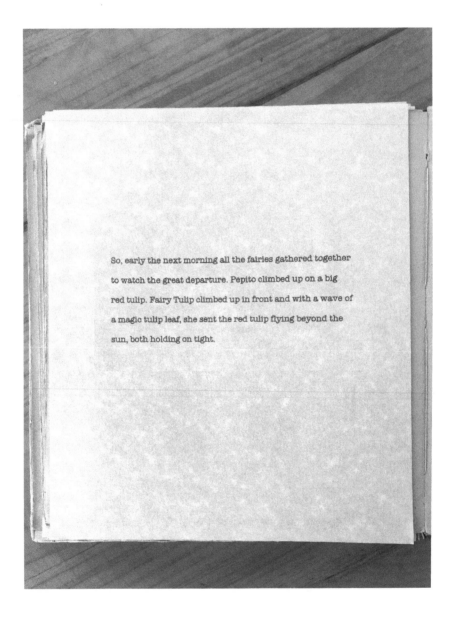

So, early the next morning all the fairies gathered together
to watch the great departure. Pepito climbed up on a big
red tulip. Fairy Tulip climbed up in front and with a wave of
a magic tulip leaf, she sent the red tulip flying beyond the
sun, both holding on tight.

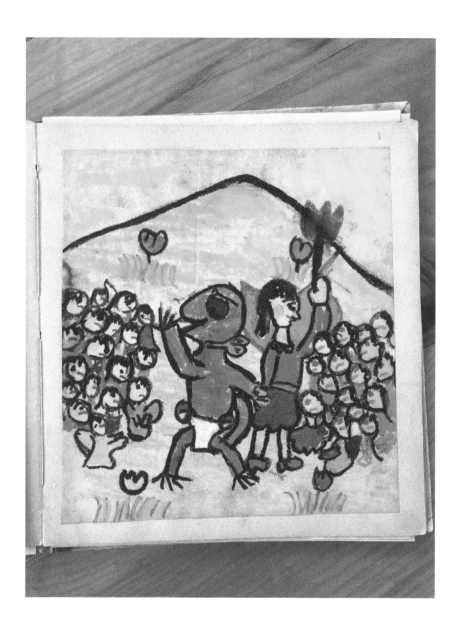

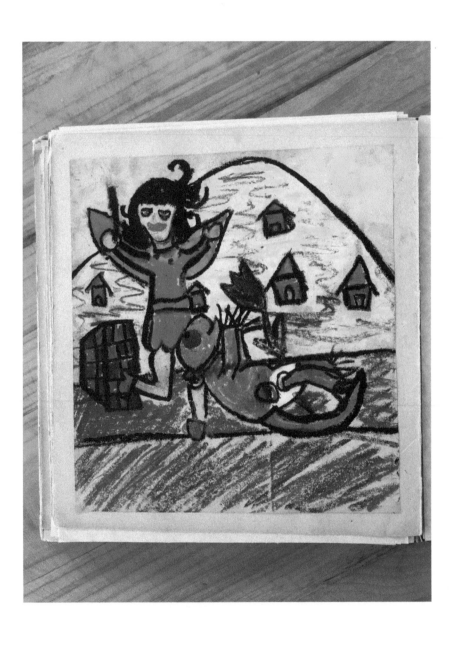

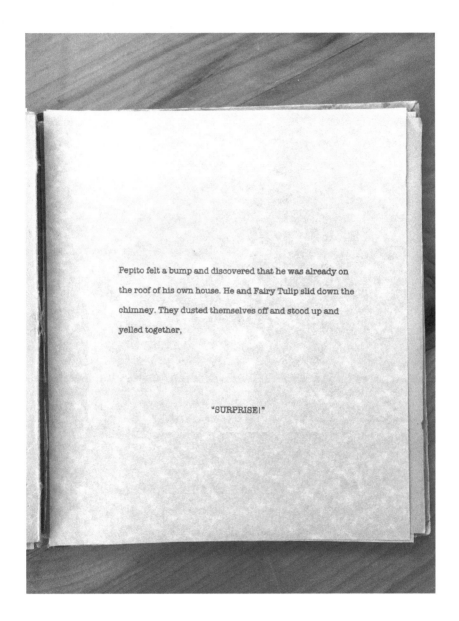

Pepito felt a bump and discovered that he was already on
the roof of his own house. He and Fairy Tulip slid down the
chimney. They dusted themselves off and stood up and
yelled together,

"SURPRISE!"

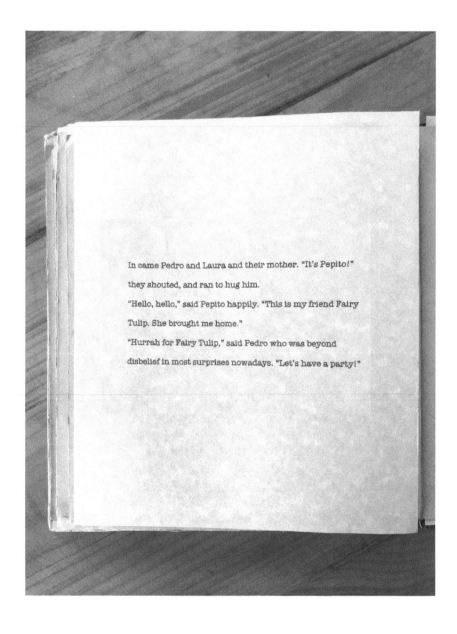

In came Pedro and Laura and their mother. "It's Pepito!"

they shouted, and ran to hug him.

"Hello, hello," said Pepito happily. "This is my friend Fairy

Tulip. She brought me home."

"Hurrah for Fairy Tulip," said Pedro who was beyond

disbelief in most surprises nowadays. "Let's have a party!"

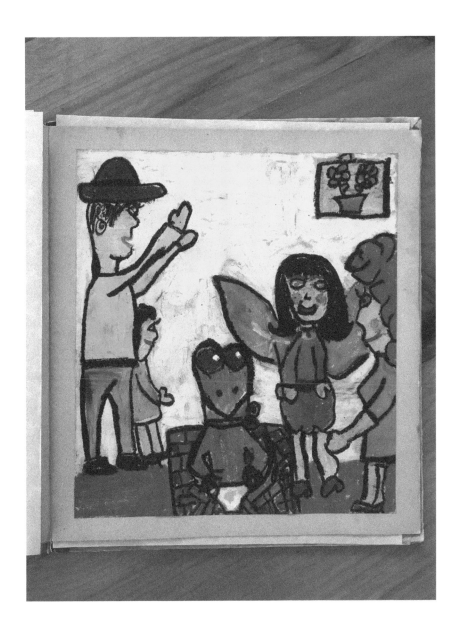

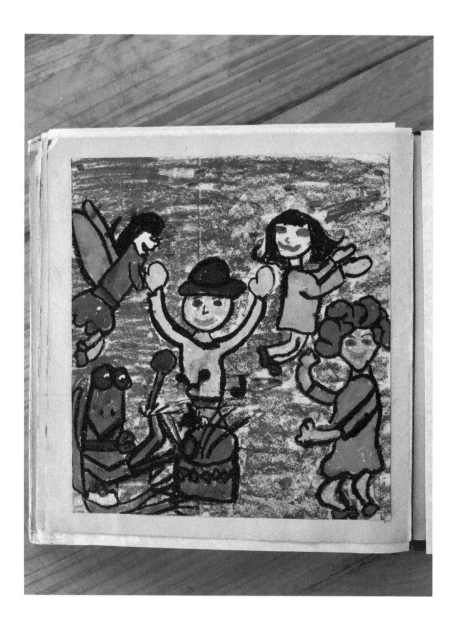

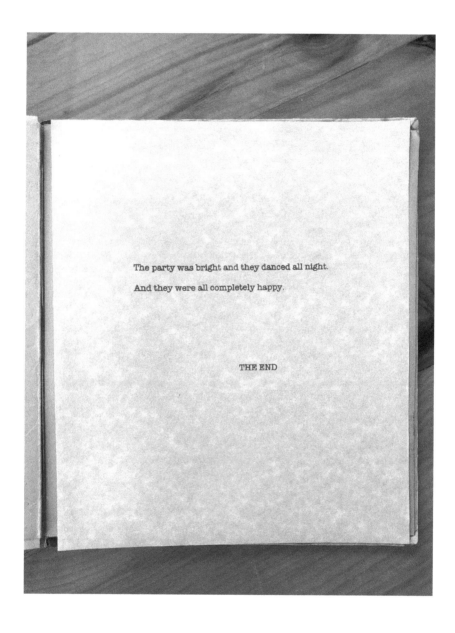

The party was bright and they danced all night.

And they were all completely happy.

THE END

CPSIA information can be obtained
at www.ICGtesting.com
Printed in the USA
LVHW070444011118
594873LV00006BA/7/P